M000303293

One, Two, What Can I Do?

Also by Connie Bergstein Dow

Dance, Turn, Hop, Learn!
Enriching Movement Activities for Preschoolers

One, Two, What Can I Do?

Dance and Music for the Whole Day

Connie Bergstein Dow

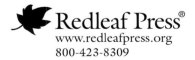
Redleaf Press®
www.redleafpress.org
800-423-8309

Published by Redleaf Press
10 Yorkton Court
St. Paul, MN 55117
www.redleafpress.org

© 2011 by Connie Bergstein Dow

All rights reserved. Unless otherwise noted on a specific page, no portion of this publication may
be reproduced or transmitted in any form or by any means, electronic or mechanical, including
photocopying, recording, or capturing on any information storage and retrieval system, without
permission in writing from the publisher, except by a reviewer, who may quote brief passages in
a critical article or review to be printed in a magazine or newspaper, or electronically transmitted
on radio, television, or the Internet.

First edition 2011
Cover design by Jim Handrigan
Cover photograph by Collage Photography
Interior typeset in Adobe Caslon and Univers and designed by Jim Handrigan
Interior photographs by Kevin Wauligman
Photographs were taken at North Avondale Montessori School and gratefully printed in this
book courtesy of North Avondale Montessori School, a magnet program in the Cincinnati
Public School system.

Printed in the U.S.A.
18 17 16 15 14 13 12 11   1 2 3 4 5 6 7 8

Library of Congress Cataloging-in-Publication Data
Bergstein Dow, Connie.
     One, two, what can I do? : dance and music for the whole day / Connie Bergstein Dow.
          p. cm.
     Summary: "This title is a collection of creative dance activities for young children. The movement
games, large-motor skill development practice, enjoyable movement problem-solving tasks, and
imaginative movement prompts come with two compact discs of delightful songs and instrumental
selections"— Provided by publisher.
     Includes bibliographical references and index.
     ISBN 978-1-60554-040-5
     1. Movement education. 2. Motor learning. 3. Dance for children. 4. Early childhood
education—Activity programs.   I. Title.
  GV452.B47 2011
  372.86—dc22
                                        2010048536

Printed on acid-free paper

For Buzz

There are short cuts to happiness, and for me dancing is one of them.
—Vicki Baum, *It Was All Quite Different*

Contents

Free-Movement Explorations

Acknowledgments

THIS BOOK has been a joy to write because of my love of dance and the opportunity to share my passion with others. I am blessed with the steadfast support I receive from my husband, Buzz, my children, David, Michael, and Jessica, and my mother, Mary Bergstein. I can always count on special friends near and far, who never fail to offer a word of encouragement, including Jane Friedman, Elaine Greiwe, Larry Hallas, Judy Hollander, Vicki Porter-Fink, Gayle Sherman, Lynn Slaughter, and Priscilla Ungers.

I turned to friend and early childhood educator Brent Reckman when I wanted to learn more about connecting children to the outdoors. I thank him for his guidance and for introducing me to author David Sobel. I also thank Carol Stromme, Special Needs Program Manager at Resources for Child Caring, for her review of the modifications that accompany each activity in the book.

I would like to thank one school and several individuals who provided me with the opportunity to present movement sessions and take photographs for this book. North Avondale Montessori School, a magnet program in the Cincinnati Public School system, hosted the photo shoot. Principal Roger Lewis, Teacher Amie Wagner, and the whole three-to-six teacher team graciously welcomed photographer Kevin Wauligman and me to their newly refurbished facility. Thank you also to Judy Naim, Adjunct Professor at Xavier University, for connecting me with the teachers at North Avondale Montessori.

Debbie Clement provided the delightful music. Music is dance's natural companion, and the book is the richer for her compositions. I give a special thanks to Mim Brodsky Chenfeld, mentor and friend, who in a moment of serendipity brought Debbie and me together, which ultimately resulted in this book and CD project.

I feel very fortunate to have worked with Redleaf Press a second time. I extend a special thank you to Redleaf Press Editor-in-Chief David Heath and Acquisitions/Development Editor Kyra Ostendorf, for believing in this book. I would like to acknowledge the hard work of Developmental Editor Laurie Herrmann, with whom I worked closely, and whose ideas and questions helped clarify and enhance the activities.

I am inspired by the creativity of fellow dancers, dance educators, early childhood professionals, and all of the adults and children whom I have had the opportunity to teach, and from whom I continue to learn.

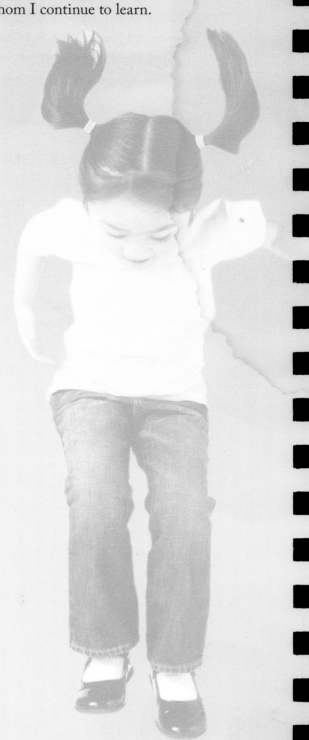

Introduction

WELCOME TO *One, Two, What Can I Do? Dance and Music for the Whole Day!* Filled with more than one hundred movement activities, this collection is your handbook to the world of dance. The activities that follow contain a wide assortment of movement ideas and musical styles to stimulate children's minds and muscles. As you explore movement with young children ages three and up, you may be surprised how versatile the activities are, how easily you can integrate dance into the learning environment, and how much fun creative movement can be.

The benefits of movement are numerous. Among the many, these are the most powerful:

- Movement enhances a child's *physical learning*.

- Movement enhances a child's *social and emotional learning*.

- Movement enhances a child's *kinesthetic learning*.

- Movement enhances a child's *cognitive learning*.

- Movement supports a teacher's *classroom management*.

Physical Learning

Movement is a physical activity. First and foremost, it addresses the way a child moves her body, learns motor skills, and develops body awareness. It also complements the natural learning style of young children, making guided movement activities the perfect forum to teach large-motor skills and refine and enhance a child's development of body control.

Exercise—Just What the Doctor Ordered

Movement, or dance (the terms are used interchangeably here and throughout the activities) is a fun physical activity—an easy way to get children up and moving. Government and health agencies are sounding the alarm about the effects of children's increasingly sedentary lifestyles.

Let's Move!, the initiative launched in 2010 by First Lady Michelle Obama, has zeroed in on a significant one: obesity.

> Over the past three decades, childhood obesity rates in America have tripled, and today, nearly one in three children in America are overweight or obese. One-third of all children born in 2000 or later will suffer from diabetes at some point in their lives; many others will face chronic obesity-related health problems like heart disease, high blood pressure, cancer, and asthma.

Teachers, parents, and caregivers are consistently encouraged to offer children opportunities to do physical activities throughout the day, with the hope that young children will establish lifelong healthy habits. How much activity is recommended? The Centers for Disease Control and many other organizations that have addressed this issue recommend children and adolescents have sixty minutes or more of physical activity each day. Invigorating dance activities can be easily integrated into a child's day, and the exercise that results will help keep young children engaged and active. *One, Two, What Can I Do?* is filled with lively, age-appropriate activities.

Physical Development—Running, Hopping, Skipping, Jumping . . .

It is important for children to participate in activities compatible with and beneficial to their physical growth and development. The U.S. Department of Health and Human Services recognizes that

> children are naturally active in an intermittent way, particularly when they do unstructured active play. During recess and in their free play and games, children use basic aerobic and bone-strengthening activities, such as running, hopping, skipping, and jumping, to develop movement patterns and skills. They alternate brief periods of moderate- and vigorous-intensity physical activity with brief periods of rest.

Dance activities offered throughout the day provide exactly this kind of outlet for children, including motor-skills development and practice, lively, playful games, and creative movement explorations.

The movement activities in this book follow the guidelines in the Position Statement of the National Association for Sport and Physical Education. The five premises of the position statement follow:

1. Teachers of young children are guides or facilitators.

   Young children learn through involvement, observation, and modeling, which requires teachers to facilitate children's active involvement in learning.

2. Children should engage in movement programs designed for their developmental levels.

   Young children need a variety of experiences that will lead to mature fundamental motor skills. . . . Teachers . . . need to fully understand the continuum of motor development.

3. Young children learn through interaction with their environment.

   Children learn through active involvement with people and objects.

4. Young children learn and develop in an integrated fashion.

   Motor, cognitive, emotional, and social development are interrelated. Learning experiences in movement should encompass and interface with other areas of development.

5. Planned movement experiences enhance play experiences.

   A combination of play along with planned movement experiences, specifically designed to help young children develop fundamental motor skills, is beneficial in assisting them in their development.

That All-Important Body Control

Children's love of movement offers teachers the opportunity to help children develop control of their bodies. While participating in guided movement activities, they learn to recognize and modulate the speed at which they are moving, and they practice starting, stopping, slowing down, and changing direction. Mastering these skills can help children acquire balance, coordination, and strength, along with the self-assurance that comes from the feeling of being in control of their bodies.

Just as important, children begin to gain awareness of others around them. Movement activities nurture spatial-awareness skills, which help children move about as a group while individually respecting the space of those around them. Group movement activities begin ideally in a personal space, or home spot, for each child. A home spot is a place to start, return to, or finish any activity. Recognizing a home spot becomes the foundation for learning to move in a shared space with others.

The concept of personal space is one that can be integrated into any group activity, from simply waiting in line to playing games on the playground. It also influences classroom management opportunities for the teacher, such as using cues to signal the cessation of activities: "Here is my stop sign—get ready to put on your brakes. Now walk slowly to your home spot, and freeze!" Directing children to focus on a task that requires body control can ease them into transitions: "Before we go to our cubbies, let's see how quietly you can stand up, and then go all the way onto your tiptoes. Now can you walk on your tiptoes to get your coat without making any noise?"

Social and Emotional Learning

Young children can learn important social and emotional skills while participating in group movement activities. The National Dance Education Organization, a research and advocacy group that studies and promotes dance and its many benefits, describes how dance can nurture social awareness in young children:

> Dance fosters social encounter, interaction, and cooperation. Children learn to communicate ideas to others through the real and immediate mode of body movement. Children quickly learn to work within a group dynamic. As the ongoing and sometimes challenging process of cooperation evolves, children learn to understand themselves in relation to others.

Social Development

Individually and as part of a group, children love the challenge of solving movement tasks while playing movement games. A movement game contains tasks and prompts to which the children respond, such as in a game of dance and freeze. When children move freely about the space, they learn to respect the others who are moving about the space with them. They listen for cues, such as when to freeze, how to stop, what shape to make with the body during the freeze. The game, which can be done in two groups, with one group watching while the other group dances, fosters the development of important social concepts, such as listening to and following instructions, cooperating in a group setting, taking turns, offering ideas, and learning to be a courteous and interested audience member.

Emotional Development and Self-Expression

Guided movement activities also offer children the opportunity to express their emotions and develop self-awareness. A movement session is a safe, controlled environment in which children have a physical outlet for processing and expressing their feelings. An activity as simple as asking the children to smile, frown, make shy, sad, or silly faces can give them the opportunity to tune in to their feelings. Dance stories, in which the children choose to move in their own ways as they interpret different situations, emotions, settings, and characters of a story, also encourage self-expression.

Creativity—Jump-Start the Imagination!

Children who can use movement as a medium for self-expression have the opportunity to explore a given topic from a different point of view—movement becomes one more tool for a child to use as he approaches a task. For instance, allowing a child to explore the question "How does a seed grow?" through words, pictures, stories, and hands-on seed planting offers valuable ways for the child to understand the concept. But what if you added the element of movement? A child can imagine himself as a tiny seed, think about the water and sunlight he needs to grow, and create his own story about what kind of plant he is as he moves through the different stages of a plant's development. Approaching learning through the medium of movement can be a powerful stimulus for creative thinking.

As young children grow up to become adults, they must be prepared to compete in the larger world. Educators understand that we must give children every opportunity to develop into innovative, original thinkers who have the ability to approach problems in many different ways. Dance and the other creative arts—drama, music, visual art, writing—offer multifaceted approaches to problem solving and can jump-start imaginations and offer new avenues for exploration.

Kinesthetic Learning

Kinesthetic learning can be one important part of the child's mastery of basic concepts. Some children may understand a concept better and more quickly if they can try it out, or physicalize it, in their own bodies. One of the guidelines of the NASPE statement for movement activities for young children points to the importance of offering them hands-on learning opportunities. Exploring ideas, relationships, emotions, stories, songs, and other themes through movement gives children the opportunity to understand different concepts through the medium of the body, reinforcing the "learning through doing" approach. Creative movement activities are the essence of kinesthetic learning.

For example, consider the concept of opposites. Children can learn the words "straight" and "crooked," they can manipulate straight and crooked objects, and they may comprehend the basic meaning of the words. But they can also experience the concept kinesthetically, or in their bodies, by making straight and curved shapes with the whole body and various body parts. They can try to move while holding their bodies in straight and crooked shapes. They can perform simple locomotor skills, such as marching and hopping, in straight and crooked floor patterns. The meaning of the opposites "straight" and "crooked" is reinforced through the kinesthetic learning.

An underlying principle of movement education is that the process is more important than the final product. A vital part of creative movement is for the child to try new movements in order to approach an idea. The child may succeed sometimes, every time, or not at all—but will certainly be moving her body in new ways while exploring solutions kinesthetically. The following concept applies throughout the activities in this book, and is a basic premise of creative movement: the exploration process and the resultant kinesthetic learning together represent the most important part of the activity.

Cognitive Learning

The strong link that exists between moving and learning may not be familiar to many people, but it is the subject of recent research yielding exciting results. This research shows that movement can actually stimulate cognition, the process of the brain's acquisition of new knowledge. This link between moving and learning makes movement a useful device for teaching almost any subject.

The Brain-Body Connection

Scientific research is shedding light on the crucial connection between moving and the learning process in both children and adults. In his book *Spark: The Revolutionary New Science of Exercise and the Brain*, John Ratey, associate professor of psychiatry at Harvard University, says exercise improves learning on three levels. It

- increases the ability to be alert, pay attention, and be motivated and ready to learn,
- readies the nerve cells and neurotransmitters to begin firing to log in and process new information, and
- prompts the development of new nerve cells.

Ratey also says:

Exercise . . . makes the brain function at its best, and in my view, this benefit of physical activity is far more important—and fascinating—than what it does for the body. Building muscles and conditioning the heart and lungs are essentially side effects. I often tell my patients that the point of exercise is to build and condition the brain.

Neurophysiologist Carla Hannaford also addresses the crucial role that movement plays in the learning process. In her book *Smart Moves: Why Learning Is Not All in Your Head*, she writes:

Movement, a natural process of life, is now understood to be essential to learning, creative thought, and high level formal reasoning. It is time to consciously bring integrative movement back into every aspect of our lives and realize, as I have, that something this simple and natural can be the source of miracles.

These studies, and the work of other researchers, are helping us understand the exciting connection between moving and learning. The results present a compelling case for parents and teachers to offer an array of movement opportunities to children.

Curriculum Enrichment

Creative dance can be integrated into almost any early childhood environment and used as a tool to stimulate learning and teach subjects across the curriculum. Movement can be axial, or stationary, and can include moving different parts of the body, going up and down from the floor to standing, turning, shaking, balancing, twisting, and hopping and jumping while staying in place. Locomotor movement takes the body from one place to another, and includes the basic motor skills of walking, marching, hopping, jumping, galloping, sliding, skipping, and leaping.

The body and its movement, then, are the raw material of dance, just as an instrument or the voice is the raw material of music. And just as the instrument utilizes the elements of melody, tempo, and rhythm to create music, the body uses the elements of space, time, and energy to create dance. When used together, these elements can generate an unlimited variety of imaginative movement ideas and make dance the versatile teaching tool it is. Virtually any subject can be taught using the medium of movement, as you will see throughout the pages of this book. *One, Two, What Can I Do?* offers activities that cross the spectrum of the curriculum, including language, mathematics, science, and social studies.

Classroom Management

For some, classroom management may be the most surprising—and the most rewarding—benefit of movement. While the idea of children dancing freely can evoke an image of them running around with no sense of control, the opposite is true. Because guided dance sessions help them develop body control, children learn to respond to your movement instructions effectively. And because movement sessions foster spatial awareness, children can respond in a productive and positive way to the guidelines and boundaries you establish for movement activities. These abilities, supported by movement, will transfer to other group situations throughout the day, especially if you offer the children reminders—"Try to stay in your home spot during circle time"—and affirm their progress—"I like how you listened to my instructions when I asked you to put on your brakes and slow down while we walk together."

Begin by using movement activities in *One, Two, What Can I Do?* as positive reinforcement for good behavior, for playful greetings and transitions, and as a break between more sedentary activities. The children will soon understand the expectations of the movement sessions and become accustomed to and comfortable with the consistent guidelines. The reward will be attentive, responsive children. Movement is well worth the effort.

Getting Started

Many adults are hesitant to introduce and use movement with groups of children, because they feel they lack the experience to do so, or because they are concerned the children will be difficult to guide. I understand their concerns, and in these activities I offer up my tried-and-true ideas developed throughout almost forty years of teaching movement to children. The activities in *One, Two, What Can I Do?* are designed to ease you into bringing movement to your early childhood environment, with clear, step-by-step directions for presenting each one. They include helpful advice for managing a group of children during an activity, ensuring the safety of the children while they move together, and maximizing the learning opportunities in all of the movement and music activities. Each activity provides instructions for how to arrange the children before you begin, which musical selections to use, how to present the activity to the children, and how to bring each session to a close. Small props may be recommended, with clear instructions about how to use them with the children, along with teaching tips for varying and enhancing the activity in the future.

The activities collected in *One, Two, What Can I Do?* are organized to reflect the different parts of the child's day.

- Part 1: Start the Day with Dance and Music offers an array of activities to use for greetings and ideas for beginning the morning routine.

- Part 2: Around the Circle contains quiet and lively circle games and exercises.

- Part 3: Transitions: Going from Here to There helps make transition time fun and creative, whether the children are going from one place to another or from one part of the day to another.

- Part 4: Group Movement Explorations consists of activities built around the basic early childhood curriculum and includes the topics of language and literacy; numbers, shapes, and patterns; science; and social studies.
- Part 5: Locomotion—Large-Motor Skill Activities is full of activities for large spaces, both indoors and outside, and includes walks and marches, slides and gallops, jumps and hops, and skips and leaps (these last two are for children ages five and up).
- Part 6: Quiet Down and Say Good-Bye offers ideas for how to help children relax and bring individual movement activities, as well as the day, to a quiet finish.
- Part 7: Dance and Music Presentation Jump-Starts is a whole array of activities that can serve as individual movement sessions or be developed into informal or more structured presentations.

Because all of the activities are divided to reflect the different parts of the young child's day, they can be plugged right into the daily routine.

Choose an Activity

The 109 activities in the book can be done in any order, and the wide variety of movement ideas allows you to find the one that is just right for you and the children in your own learning environment. After reviewing the part and activity titles and descriptions, as well as the indexes, you can choose an activity based on the space available, the musical selection, or the subject matter. You will enjoy discovering the nature of each activity and selecting the movement that fits your needs at any time.

One, Two, What Can I Do? lies flat for ease of use while guiding the children through the activities. Once you have chosen the activity that fits your needs, you can hold the book open, or position it nearby, so you can glance at the script as you move through the lesson.

Any Space Will Do

A common misconception about movement is that a large space is necessary. No one will argue that a big, unobstructed space isn't ideal, but movement sessions can be done in a space that accommodates the group standing or sitting in a circle, in a home spot, or walking in a line for a transition. In fact, sometimes working in a limited space generates interesting and creative ideas for movement that would be different if a larger space were available. The important message is that you can bring movement to children in any space, large or small, indoors or outside. You will find lots of activities in *One, Two, What Can I Do?* that will work in the space that is available to you.

No matter what shape or size space you will use to present movement activities to children, it is helpful to prepare your space ahead of time. Clear the area as much as possible to keep it safe and to avoid distractions. Create visual boundaries for the movement session, such as a large rug laid out flat or classroom chairs turned away. Be sure to point out the boundaries to the children before they start moving. Allow them to walk around in the designated area and choose their home spots or find their assigned spots so they have a place to begin, are oriented to the spatial boundaries, and are ready to listen to instructions. Designate boundaries when dancing outdoors too.

If you incorporate movement into the daily routine without making a separate movement space as described above, then the choice of activities you present is the most important factor in accommodating your space. Many of the activities in this collection work well in small or obstructed spaces. For the times when a large, open area, such as a gym, is available, you will find a number of activities devoted specifically to large-motor skills. And many of the activities work well outside. Information regarding the ideal space required for an activity is noted in each activity's "What You Need" section as well as in the indexes.

Guide the Movement

An important component of this collection is the teacher's script. Many books about movement offer ideas for activities but don't give precise information to the teacher about how to guide the children through the session. *One, Two, What Can I Do?* provides scripts for the adult to use throughout the activity, with suggestions for prompting the children as they explore each new idea. The script is an outline of the basic structure of each movement activity, with suggested spoken directions given in boldface. While you guide the activities, allow the children time to develop the ideas presented in the script. For example, instructions of two or three sentences in the script could take five to ten minutes, if you allow each new idea to develop, with different children approaching the ideas in unique ways. The children will have many creative and interesting solutions to the movement prompts, which can lead the activity in new and imaginative directions. Along the same lines, you may want to add your own ideas and variations. You can set the pace and boundaries within which the activities and variations unfold, while allowing the children's imaginations to soar.

Color photographs of children participating in creative movement activities are interspersed throughout the book. The photographs illustrate children exploring individual responses to various movement prompts, and solving them in unique ways. It is important to reiterate here a central theme present throughout the book: there is no single or correct response or solution to a movement task or prompt. The questions and ideas in the activities will elicit movement responses from the children, and this process in itself is the essence of the learning that takes place. Moving their bodies in new ways while thinking creatively about the way to solve tasks is the learning process, which is a valuable part of the movement experience for children. The photographs illustrate children responding with a wide variety of movement ideas as they participate in different activities.

Move to the Music

Music provides children with many of the same benefits as creative movement—and some others as well. Music nurtures early language and reasoning skills, with its rhythm, rhymes, patterns, and words. It provides another arena for stimulating children's creativity and imagination. Like movement, music is a means for self-expression. Virtually any subject can be taught or reinforced through music; the repetition of the words of a song alone can be a wonderful teaching tool.

Many of the activities in *One, Two, What Can I Do?* were designed to be enjoyed along with specific musical selections, which are indicated at the beginning of each lesson. Music adds a delightful dimension to the movement activities, and it reinforces the learning that takes place. When movement and music are both incorporated into the children's greetings, transitions, circle times, and quiet-down and good-bye activities, the combination can increase the fun and perhaps make an activity a familiar favorite in the daily routine. Two CDs of those vocal and instrumental selections by arts enrichment specialist Debbie Clement are included in this movement collection. You will be delighted with the wide variety of child-friendly songs and instrumentals that make up the recordings.

Use Auditory and Visual Cues

Whether or not music is suggested with an activity, it is helpful to have handy a small drum or tambourine. Use it to keep the beat when needed and to supply an auditory cue to the children. You can also use your hands and your voice to clap and sing out cues to create the rhythmic structure for the movement session.

Auditory and visual cues—for example, flicking the lights on and off, or holding up a large prop or picture, such as a stop sign or stoplight—are very helpful during movement time. The use of cues aids in establishing a familiar routine that immediately directs the children's attention. Tapping a small drum or tambourine, holding up a sign, or even coming up with your own specific vocal or visual cue can be used as a signal for the children to return to the home spot, to prepare for new instructions, or to stop or freeze. Guidelines for using the auditory and visual cues are included in the activity descriptions.

Modifications to Keep Every Child Dancing

Dance and music are often used to reach children whose learning styles are best addressed in less traditional ways. Movement sessions are especially beneficial to children with special needs, because they provide another avenue for learning and self-expression. For example, children with high energy levels, who may have difficulty focusing for long periods of time, can benefit from guided movement activities because they provide a positive outlet for the release of excess energy. At the same time, teachers can use movement to help children channel their energy into rich learning opportunities. *One, Two, What Can I Do?* offers specific ideas for including all children in the dance and music sessions. There is almost always a way to adapt a movement to suit a child's abilities.

When teaching movement to all children, it is important to remember the foundation on which creative dance is built: the kinesthetic learning that happens as a result of the exploration is the crux of the movement experience. No matter what the activity, the process of doing the movement is more important than the skill level at which a child performs the movement. This tenet is what allows creative movement to be inclusive of all learning styles, even those of children who may have a hearing or vision impairment, or whose ability to move is limited.

Modifications for children with special needs are included with each activity. Use these ideas to encourage all children to move to the best of their abilities. Study the suggestions for adaptations before you begin the activity, and integrate your own ideas based on the individual situation of the child. The extra time and effort it may take to include all children will create fun and valuable learning opportunities for those who might otherwise be excluded from the movement session.

Dance Outdoors

The philosophy of creative dance—encouraging kinesthetic learning, exploration, and curiosity—lends itself well to the growing movement of reconnecting children with the outdoors. Noted author and educator David Sobel describes the importance of children's connection with nature:

> Empathy between the child and the natural world should be a main objective for children ages four through seven. As children begin their forays into the natural world, we can encourage feelings for the creatures living there. Early childhood is characterized by a lack of differentiation between the self and the other. Children feel implicitly drawn to baby animals; a child feels pain when someone else scrapes her knee. Rather than force separateness, we want to cultivate that sense of connectedness so that it can become the emotional foundation for the more abstract ecological concept that everything is connected to everything else. Stories, songs, moving like animals, celebrating seasons, and fostering Rachel Carson's "sense of wonder" should be primary activities during this stage.

> Cultivating relationships with animals, both real and imagined, is one of the best ways to foster empathy during early childhood. Children want to run like deer, to slither along the ground like snakes, to be clever as a fox and quick like a bunny.

Many of the movement activities in *One, Two, What Can I Do?* can be done outdoors, and there are a number that pertain to nature and animals. Playful games, stories, poems, and other explorations spark the child's imagination and teach him about weather, life cycles, animal behavior and characteristics, and other important concepts about the natural world. See the indexes to find the "movement in nature" activity you are looking for.

Let's Move!

Moving is what children do the minute they begin each day. It is natural and fun, and one of the primary ways children learn about their surroundings. I hope teachers and caregivers will use *One, Two, What Can I Do?* to explore creative dance with children, and in so doing, reap the many benefits of this joyful art form.

References

Centers for Disease Control and Prevention. 2011. "Physical Activity for Everyone." Accessed January 16. http://www.cdc.gov/physicalactivity/everyone/guidelines/ children.html

Hannaford, Carla. 1995. *Smart Moves: Why Learning Is Not All in Your Head.* Arlington, VA: Great Ocean Publishers, 214.

Let's Move! America's Move to Raise a Healthier Generation of Kids. 2010. "Learn the Facts." Accessed January 16. http://www.letsmove.gov/learnthefacts.php.

National Association for Sport and Physical Education. 2000. Appropriate Practices in Movement Programs for Young Children Ages 3–5.

National Dance Education Organization. 2011. Standards for Dance in Early Childhood. Accessed January 16. http://www.ndeo.org.

Ratey, John J. 2008. *Spark: The Revolutionary New Science of Exercise and the Brain.* New York: Little, Brown, 53, 3.

Sobel, David. 1998. "Beyond Ecophobia." Accessed January 16. http://www .yesmagazine.org/issues/education-for-life/803. Adapted from volume one of the Orion Society Nature Literacy Series, *Beyond Ecophobia: Reclaiming the Heart in Nature Education.*

U.S. Department of Health & Human Services. 2008. Physical Activity Guidelines for Americans. Accessed January 16. http://www.health.gov/paguidelines/ guidelines/

START THE DAY WITH DANCE AND MUSIC

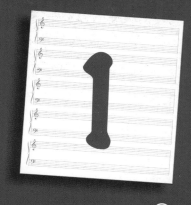

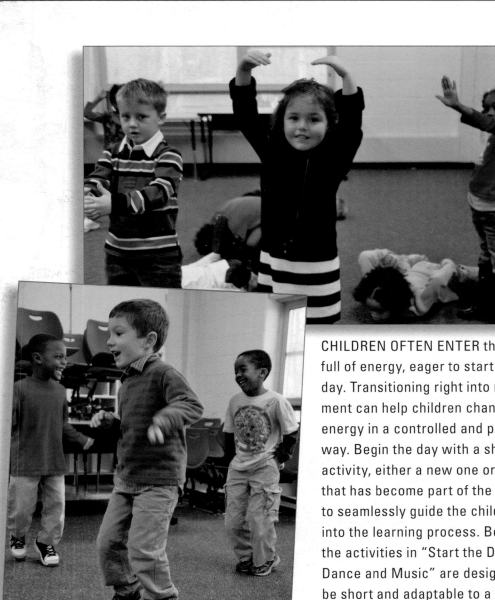

CHILDREN OFTEN ENTER the room full of energy, eager to start the day. Transitioning right into movement can help children channel their energy in a controlled and positive way. Begin the day with a short activity, either a new one or one that has become part of the routine, to seamlessly guide the children into the learning process. Because the activities in "Start the Day with Dance and Music" are designed to be short and adaptable to a small area—and many are suitable for outdoors—most do not require musical accompaniment.

High Five

. . . .

1

Once the children learn the words and movement to this activity, "High Five" can be used to greet the children, one by one, as they come into the room or as a group activity to begin the daily routine.

What You Need

☼ a small space, indoors or outside

What You Do

Begin with the children standing in a circle or a line. Say the rhyme aloud to the children, and then ask them to say it with you.

High Five

**High five
Low five
Clapping fives
Jumps and jives**

Now repeat it again, slowly, while you perform the movements with the words. Do this several times with the children until they can say the words and do the movements at the same time.

High five

- stand on tiptoe with your hand held up for a high five

Low five

- stoop low with your hand held down for a low five

Clapping fives

- clap your hands three times

Jumps and jives

- jump three times

After the children have repeated "High Five" several times, finish the activity by having them freeze in the high-five position.

Modifications

The words to this movement activity can easily be changed to accommodate children's different needs. For example, the word "jumps" can be changed to "jiggles" for a child who cannot jump, and then the activity can be performed in a sitting position.

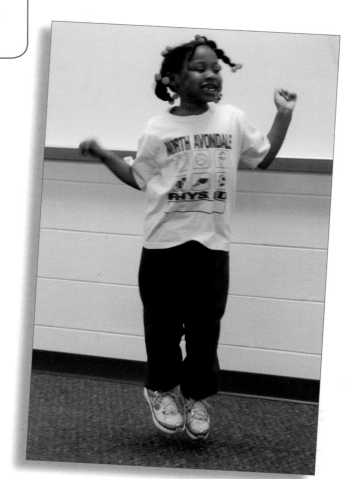

No-Hands Shake

• • • • • • • • • • • • •

2

"No-Hands Shake" is a problem-solving activity. Problem-solving activities can spur creativity and challenge the child to come up with a movement solution to a question, task, or prompt. Guide the children through the task so that they each "answer" with an individual kinesthetic response to the prompt. For a group problem-solving movement task, follow up with Activity 3: Our Special Greeting.

What You Need

☼ small space, indoors or outside

What You Do

Have the children sit or stand in a line or circle. Say to the children:

When we meet someone, we often greet that person by shaking his or her hand, don't we? Well, we're going to think of a new way to greet someone. Let's pretend we're meeting one another for the first time. Each of you will make up a new no-hands shake, and one by one, I will do that new no-hands shake with you. Will you do a shoulder shake? A head shake? A foot shake? Let's see how many different ways we can greet each other!

Walk around the circle or down the line so you can engage each child one by one. A child may try to shake your hand, but remind her that this is a "no-hands" shake and offer, for example, your elbow instead. Once you have done an "elbow shake" (to do this, shake your elbow near but not touching the child's elbow) with the first child, the others will get the idea. You can continue to prompt with other body parts—your head, eyes, tongue, wrist, upper back, knee, side of the body, toes, backside, or leg.

2

Finish the activity by saying to the children:

Let's all shake the one part of our body we chose for our no-hands shake! We'll do this all together for a few counts. Hold a low shape when I say, "Freeze!"

Modifications

This is a good activity for a child who may have trouble using her body in certain ways, because there are so many solutions, or different parts of the body, to use for the no-hands shake. For example, a child can use his upper body only, or even just his eyelids, to perform the no-hands shake.

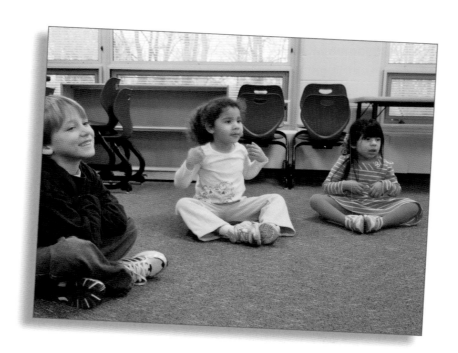

Our Special Greeting

"Our Special Greeting" is a group problem-solving activity. The solution to the movement task will be generated using ideas from the children as a result of questions you ask them. Then all of the children will perform the group greeting together.

What You Need

☼ a small space, indoors or outside

What You Do

Ask the children to stand in a line or circle and place yourself where they can all see you clearly. If you want the children to develop a seated movement greeting, have them sit in a line or circle. Say to the children:

Wouldn't it be fun to have our own special greeting? Let's think about how to do this. I think the greeting should have three parts. It should have:

- **a gesture—for example, a thumbs up, a head pat, or an elbow flap**

- **a noise—for example, clapping, stomping, or voicing a funny sound**

- **a finishing position—for example, sit down, freeze in an "X" shape, or jump high and land in a specific position**

With the children, discuss what gesture, noise, and finishing position the special greeting will have and how many times you will do each one. Then say to the children:

Now that we've chosen the three parts of our special greeting, let's put them all together. We'll try it a few times as a group. Then I'll walk

3

down the line and do the greeting with each of you individually. After that, we'll do our special greeting one more time, all together.

Combining some of the examples from above, your special greeting might be:

- two elbow flaps

- three stomps

- a jump up into the air, freezing with two "thumbs up" when you land

Modifications

Encourage children with different abilities to contribute ideas, so the group greeting is one in which all children can participate. When a child comes up with a movement idea, encourage all of the children to respond as they are able. For example, if the group has expressed that it would like the special greeting to end in a jump and then finish in the shape of a hug, some of the children may prefer to throw their arms into the air instead, and then hug themselves in the ending shape along with the group.

The children may want to think up a new special greeting each day, create their own unique individual greeting, or use this particular one day after day.

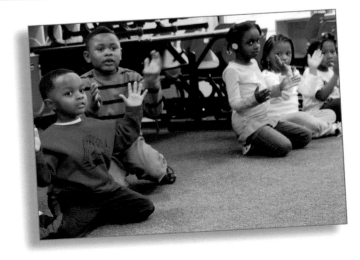

Morning Rap

· · · · · · · · · · ·

4

"Morning Rap" is a rhythm and rhyme game with movements and can be used to teach children about song structure: chorus, verse, chorus. Once the children have learned the rap and its structure (first the verse, then the chorus, then the next verse), along with the corresponding movements, it will be a fun activity for them to do day after day.

What You Need

☼ a small space, indoors or outside

What You Do

Have the children stand side by side in a line. If the group is large, ask the children to stagger the lines, making sure everyone can see you clearly. Say the "Morning Rap" chorus aloud several times until the children can say the words with you. Begin to do the movements while you say the chorus, and have the children try the movements while they rap along with you.

Morning Rap Chorus

Step, clap, step, clap, step, clap

- sidestep to one side and clap while you say these words

Do the morning rap!

- stand in place, bend knees, form loose fists with your hands, and make small circles with your hands in front of your body

Step, clap, step, clap, step, clap

- sidestep to the other side and clap while you say these words

4

Do the morning rap!

- stand in place, bend knees, form loose fists with your hands, and make small circles with your hands in front of your body

Add the following verses one by one. The verses can be added slowly—one new one per day or one new one per week—until the children know the whole rap. There are no set movements for the verses, so the children can clap and move freely in place. Repeat the chorus with its movements between each verse.

Well here I am, I'm ready for the day.
I'll see my friends, we like to play.

How are you? I am fine.
I hope you like my morning rhyme!

Isn't it fun to dance and move?
I love to dance and move and groove!

We can step and clap and bop.
We will dance 'til we're ready to stop!

Finish with the last verse. Then say, "Flop!" and the children can fall into a floppy shape while standing, or flop all the way to the floor.

You can use the "Morning Rap" chorus as a way to begin to teach right and left.

Modifications

A child can play a small percussion instrument and move any parts of her body that she is able while she raps the words.

Say "Welcome" with Your Whole Body!

"Say 'Welcome' with Your Whole Body!" helps children distinguish the two syllables in the word "welcome." The idea of the two distinct sounds is then used as the basis for creating different movements.

What You Need

☼ a small space

☼ "Shine & Brighten" instrumental (disc 2, track 37)

What You Do

Have the children stand in a home spot. Say to the children:

The word "welcome" has two different sounds. Can you hear them when I say the word slowly? "Wel" and "come." Can you say the two sounds with me? Now let's say "welcome" together with our voices: "Welcome!"

Next let's think of ways other parts of our bodies can say welcome. Just as there are two sounds in the word "welcome," we'll make a welcome movement in two parts. Let's start with our heads. How can we make two different movements with our heads? Nod your head up and down or shake your head side to side, for example. The children can follow your example or think of other ways to move their heads, such as tilting an ear toward a shoulder. The children can do their own movements, or you can choose which ones the group will use together.

Continue through all the body parts: shoulders, arms, hands, upper torso, hips, legs, feet, and whole body, performing two distinct movements with

5

each body part, and then the whole body. Once you have finished that part of the activity, lead the children through all of the different movements they have come up with, one after another. The progression of body-part movements becomes a welcome dance. Perform the welcome dance to music—play "Shine & Brighten" instrumental!

Modifications

Children can also participate in this activity seated in a home spot. If there is a body part they have difficulty moving, such as their legs, invite them to come up with more movements for their arms. Encourage them to do the arm movements while other children are moving their legs.

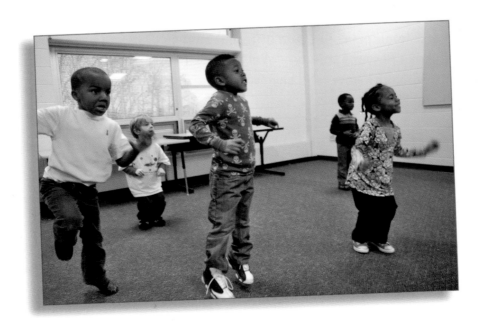

Sun Is Rising

"Sun Is Rising" is a short rhyme with accompanying movements. It can be used to greet the day and to lead into other "beginning of the day" routines.

What You Need

☼ a small space

What You Do

Begin with the children sitting in a circle or a line with a full arm's length between each child. Say the rhyme aloud line by line, asking the children to repeat it after you.

Sun Is Rising

Sun is rising in the sky.
Midday now, it's very high.
Feel the warmth, close your eyes.
Every day the sun will rise!

Now repeat it slowly once again, this time performing the movements with the words. Do this several times until the children can say the words and do the movements at the same time.

Sun is rising in the sky.

- sitting with your legs crossed, make a circle in front of your body with your arms, about chest high

Midday now, it's very high.

- make a circle overhead with your arms

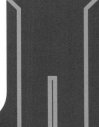

6

Feel the warmth, close your eyes.

- begin to open your arms and lower them until they are out to your sides with your palms up, your face tilting up, and your eyes closed

Every day the sun will rise!

- let your arms float down to the floor to rest by the sides of your legs, open your eyes, and gaze straight ahead, returning to the starting position

Repeat the movement activity several times.

Modifications

Children may sit on chairs or in wheelchairs or stand for this activity. For children who are hearing impaired or deaf, draw a picture in four parts, and point them out as you teach the movements: (1) a rising sun, (2) a sun high in the sky, (3) a face looking up with eyes closed, and (4) the rising sun again (picture 1).

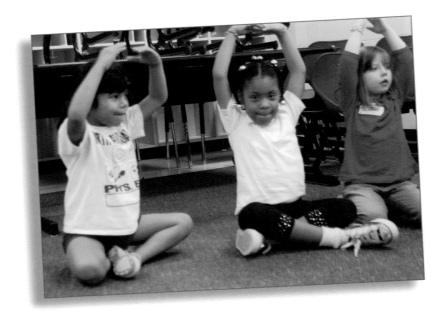

Good Morning, Fingers! ¡Buenos Días, Dedos!

7

In "Good Morning, Fingers! ¡Buenos Días, Dedos!" a counting game, use small- or large-movement variations depending on the size of the space available to you. Saying the verse in Spanish adds a fun and enriching element.

What You Need

☼ a small space

☼ finger puppets (optional; cut the fingers off of an old pair of gloves and write a number, one through ten, on each of the cut-off fingers)

What You Do

Have each child stand in a home spot with enough room to perform the various movements. If your space is limited, have the children stand in a circle. Say to the children:

Let's say good morning to our fingers! First we'll say the rhyme in English, and then we'll say the rhyme in Spanish. Count along on your fingers as we say each number.

How Many Fingers?

**One, two, three,
Four, five, six,
Seven, eight, nine,
Ten fingers mine!**

Now let's try it in Spanish!

1

¿Cuántos Dedos?

Uno, dos, tres,
Cuatro, cinco, seis,
Siete, ocho, nueve,
¡Yo tengo diez!

Let's get our fingers dancing! Now when we say the rhyme in English, let's stretch our bodies, reach our arms to the sky, and wiggle our fingers up high.

Now let's crouch down low and count our fingers in Spanish.

This time, can you stand tall and turn slowly around while you say the rhyme in English?

Now let's turn slowly in the other direction while we say the rhyme in Spanish.

Next let's bounce our bodies by gently bending our knees. Let's do this while we say the rhyme first in English and then in Spanish.

Let's finish by saying the rhyme in English while we jump, and then we'll jump while we say it in Spanish.

Now that we're finished, let's thank our fingers for dancing: Thank you, fingers! ¡Gracias, dedos! Can you make your fingers take a bow while you say "thank you" and "gracias"?

Modifications

If any of the children have speech limitations, you can carefully verbalize the numbers while the children perform the movements only. Encourage them to gradually begin to repeat the numbers with you as they continue to do the movements. Do not try the Spanish verse until the children are comfortable saying the numbers in English.

Weather Greetings and a Weather Dance

8

The weather greetings will help children identify the day's weather, and the weather dance will help them learn a movement sequence as individual movements are added each day. "Weather Greetings and a Weather Dance" will be the greeting for five consecutive mornings. Repeat this activity during all sorts of weather—sunny, stormy, windy, or cloudy, for example—so you can utilize all the movements in the weather dance.

What You Need

☼ a small space

☼ "Sunscreen" (disc 1, track 12)

☼ a weekly weather chart

What You Do

For each day's weather greeting and weather dance, have the children stand in a home spot spread throughout the space. Make sure they all can see the weather chart from their spots.

The weather, weather movements, and sound effects that follow are suggestions. The children may enjoy making up their own.

On the first day, say to the children:

What's the weather today? Yes, it's sunny! Let's greet the day by doing our movement for sunny weather. Do the sunny-weather movement several times with the children.

On the second day, say:

What's the weather today? Cloudy! Let's do our weather movement for a cloudy day. Do the cloudy-weather movement several times with the children.

Now combine the first day's sunny-weather movement and the second day's cloudy-weather movement, and repeat the movements one after the other several times with the children. Say to them:

Do you remember what the weather was yesterday? Let's look at the weather chart to help us remember. It was sunny, that's right. Now let's do yesterday's weather movement, and then let's do today's weather movement right after it.

For each remaining day of the activity, select and practice a weather movement. After you've practiced the new day's weather movement, review the previous days' movements. Put the sequence of movements together and rehearse it with the children. By Friday, the weather dance will be a progression of movements—your weather dance. Repeat the weather dance several times with the children to help them remember the sequence. Then do the weather dance with the music "Suncreen." Ask the children to freeze at the end of the music in a shape that reminds them of their favorite weather.

Sunny-Weather Movement

Stand and hold your arms down in front of your body in the shape of a circle. Let your fingertips touch or nearly touch. Use your arms to show the sun's rising and setting by lifting the circle to your left, raising it up over your head, lowering it down to your right, and then returning it to the starting position. Let the upper body follow as the arms delineate a large circle. Add a "Whee!" sound as you do the circular movement.

Cloudy-Weather Movement

Let your arms relax at your sides. Then, as if fluffing big cottony clouds, billow your arms out to the side several times as you slowly turn around. Make gentle puffing sounds along with the movement.

Rainy-Weather Movement

While standing, raise your arms overhead and go up on tiptoe. Slowly lower your arms as you wiggle your fingers. As you lower your arms, lower your body as you go from tiptoe to a low crouch. Make a drip-drop sound with your voice to go along with the rain movements.

Stormy-Weather Movement

The movement for stormy weather is just like the movement for rainy weather. Perform the movements more energetically and dramatically and add sound effects, such as saying "crash" and "boom" to simulate the sound of thunder.

Windy-Weather Movement

Leading with your arms, wave arms and body in a side-to-side swaying motion. The arms and body should feel relaxed as you gently sway first to one side and then to the other. Add sound effects, such as a whooshing noise, to create the wind.

Snowy-Weather Movement

Stand and slowly turn around in a circle as you alternate bending and straightening your knees. Gently shake your fingers in all directions while you slowly turn your body around in a circle. Because snow falls so quietly, make this a peaceful, silent movement.

An important reminder as you present this activity to young children is that learning and sequencing movement is a process and does not necessarily lead to a finished product. Getting the children to repeat exact movements in an exact order is not nearly as important as creating an environment for the children to explore new movements and begin to understand the idea of sequencing. In the free dance, encourage the children to use the weather movements as a starting point, but allow them to use their

Modifications

These movements can be changed and adapted; the ideas provided for each weather pattern are only guidelines. You and the children might prefer to come up with your own weather movements and sounds. Some children may be better able to perform the movements seated, doing the body, arm, and head movements only for each weather variation.

creativity and imaginations to try other movements as well. Prompts such as, "What do you like to do in rainy weather? Do you like to stomp in mud puddles?" can help stimulate movement ideas for the free dance.

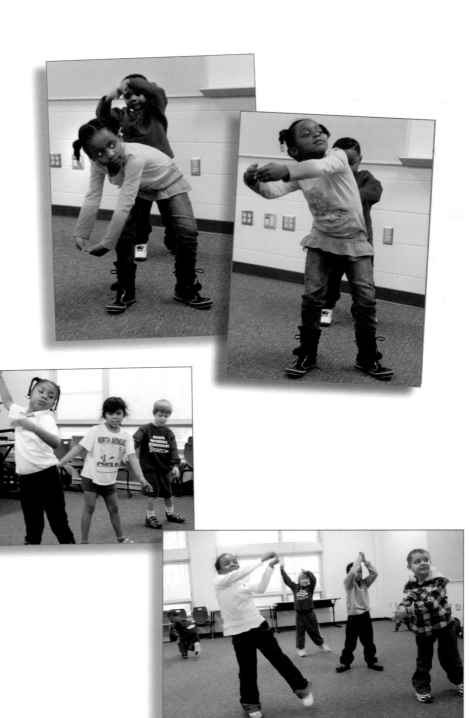

Happy Face

9

"Happy Face" is a playful forum for children to think about and acknowledge different feelings. The game maintains an upbeat tone and finishes with a delightful song about feeling happy.

What You Need

☼ a small space

☼ "Happy Face" (disc 1, track 6)

What You Do

To begin, seat the children in a line or circle. Allow them to move about the room during the free dance. Say to the children:

Let's begin by thinking about different feelings. What face do you wear when you are happy? Now let's try sad. What does your face do when you are sad? What do your arms do? How about mad? Silly? Shy? Scared? Now let's make our happy faces again.

I'm going to put on some music about happy faces. Play "Happy Face." **Let's stand up, move around the room, and dance to the music. Think about other things we do when we're happy. Do you hug yourself? Do you like to jump? Do you clap your hands? What else?**

As we dance about being happy, let's not use our voices. Let's use just our faces and our body movements to show that we're happy as we dance to this fun song. When the music is finished, freeze in a happy or silly shape.

Modifications

The child with autism can participate in all of the movements. In order to help him understand the instructions, bring or draw simple pictures of faces with different emotions and hold them up during the corresponding verbal instructions.

[37]

"Hello!" in Many Languages

10

"'Hello!' in Many Languages" is based on the song "Jambo: Hello," which teaches us how to say "hello" in Swahili, Spanish, German, French, and Japanese. "'Hello!' in Many Languages" can be the greeting for five consecutive mornings, and the children will learn five new ways to say "hello." Activity 11: Jambo: Hello is a longer circle activity that supplements the learning in this greeting activity. For pronunciation of the foreign words, listen to "Jambo: Hello."

What You Need

☼ a small space

☼ "Jambo: Hello" (disc 1, track 7) (optional)

What You Do

Day 1

As each child enters the room, greet her with a wave and say, "Jambo, hello!" Once all the children have entered the room, ask them to say "jambo" to each other, waving their hands as they say it. Then explain that "jambo" is the way children who speak Swahili greet each other.

Day 2

As each child enters the room, greet him with a wave and say, "Hola"—"hello" in Spanish. Once all the children have entered the room, ask them to say "hola" to each other and to wave, just as they did with "jambo" on day 1. Explain that this is the way children who speak Spanish say "hello."

Day 3

As each child enters the room, greet her with a wave and say the German "guten Tag!" Once all the children have entered the room, ask them to say "guten Tag!" to each other and to wave, just as they did with "hola" on day 2. "Guten Tag" is the way to say "hello" in German!

Day 4

As each child enters the room, greet him with a wave and say, "Bonjour!" Once all the children have entered the room, ask them to say "bonjour" to each other and to wave, just as they did with "guten Tag" on day 3. "Bonjour" is the way French-speaking children greet one another.

Day 5

As each child enters the room, greet her with a wave and say the Japanese "konnichiwa!" Once all the children have entered the room, ask them to say "konnichiwa" to each other and to wave, just as they did with "bonjour" on day 4. "Konnichiwa" is the word for "hello" in Japanese.

Once the children have greeted one another on day 5, review with the children each of the day's greetings and the languages they represent. Wave to each other as you and the children repeat each of the greetings. Now you may proceed to Activity 11: Jambo: Hello.

Modifications

Sign language can be used when "hello" is said in each of the different languages.

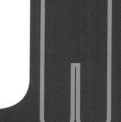

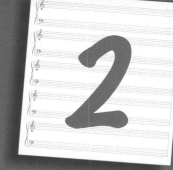

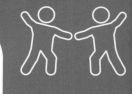

AROUND THE CIRCLE

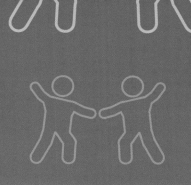

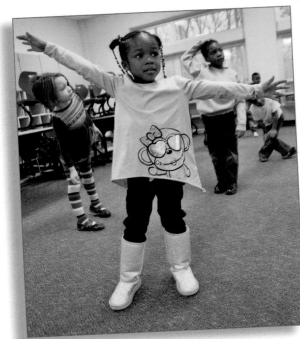

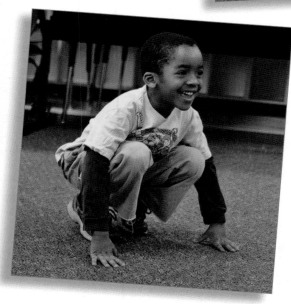

MOVEMENT can be an excellent vehicle for reinforcing important circle time concepts. These concepts can include working cooperatively, sharing ideas, taking turns, reviewing and reinforcing the daily routine, and helping each child feel included in the group. The activities in "Around the Circle" are designed for a space that will accommodate the children sitting or standing in a circle with enough room between each child so the movement of others is not impeded.

Jambo: Hello!

"Jambo: Hello!" reinforces the learning of the greetings in different languages by creating a movement to go with each one and including a song as accompaniment. The greetings in each of the five languages are repeated several times in the song. "Jambo: Hello!" is a follow-up to Activity 10: "Hello!" in Many Languages, although it can also stand alone.

What You Need

☼ a small space (the free dance at the end of the activity can be done in place in the circle or by moving throughout the shared space)

☼ "Jambo: Hello" (disc 1, track 7)

☼ a world map

What You Do

Ask the children to sit in a circle. Remind them that "hello" is the word we say to greet one another, and help them remember the other ways they learned to say "hello" in Activity 10: "jambo," "hola," "guten Tag," "bonjour," and "konnichiwa." Using a world map, point to the different countries when you explain where the greetings are spoken.

Now play a hello game using the music "Jambo: Hello." Play the music once so the children are familiar with the song. When you play it a second time, explain to the children that you want them to wave each time they hear one of the hello words. But instead of waving with their hands, encourage them to come up with a different kind of waving. For example:

• **When you hear the word "jambo," you can wave with your foot!**

• **When you hear the word "hola," you can wave with your head!**

• **When you hear "guten Tag," try waving with your elbow!**

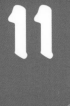

- **When you hear "bonjour," wave with your upper body!**

- **When you hear "konnichiwa," you can wave with as many body parts as you can at the same time!**

Review the five waves a couple of times, and then play the music. Encourage the children to sing the words to the song in addition to doing the movements to reinforce learning the words.

Now ask the children to stand up and do a free dance to the same music. They can dance in place or move about the room. Remind the children of the different kinds of waves they've already tried, and ask them if they can think of more ways to wave and greet each other while dancing.

Modifications

The body parts for waving can be chosen according to the unique needs of the children. If a child is very limited in her movement, she can blink her eyes or flutter her fingers for her greeting.

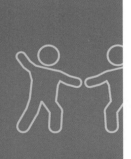

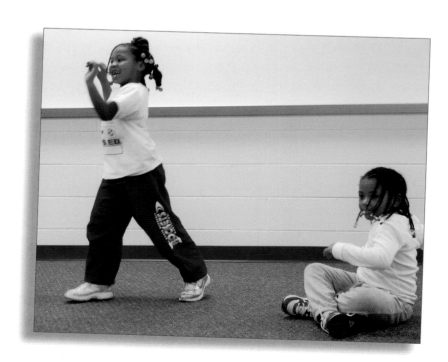

Wake Up, Muscles!

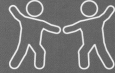

"Wake Up, Muscles!" can be used as a warm-up to begin the day. It is a great way to ease into more lively activities and to introduce children to the idea of warming up the body before exercising. Activity 64: Muscle Mania is a good follow-up activity.

What You Need

☼ a small space

☼ a muscle chart (optional) and a resistance band or a strip of stretchy fabric

What You Do

Have the children sit in a circle, with enough room between each other to stretch out arms and legs. Say to the children:

Let's begin by talking about something in our bodies that helps us move. We can help make these things stronger by walking, jumping, climbing, dancing, and doing many other fun activities and exercises. Can you guess what I'm talking about? Muscles! Muscles help us move our body parts in many different ways, and you can help make your muscles strong and healthy by staying active. Look at this chart to see how many muscles we have in our bodies. If you do not have a muscle chart, skip this comment and move on to the next one.

Our muscles can be both strong and stretchy at the same time, just like this resistance band. Our muscles can stretch like this! Let each child have a chance to feel the band or strip of fabric as you stretch it. **Do you like to stretch your body in the morning when you wake up? What parts of your body do you stretch?**

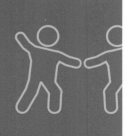

12

Let's do some stretches together. Let's imagine we're just waking up in the morning. We're still feeling tired, and we need to do something that will make us feel energetic! Gently rub your eyes, stretch your arms upward, and yawn with your mouth open wide. Open and close your eyes, and open and close your mouth. Stick out your tongue and move it from side to side. Move your head up and down and from side to side. Wave good morning to your friends across the circle.

Now stand up and wave as big as you can while you stretch your arms high and stand on your tiptoes. Come down from your tiptoes, and put your hands on your hips and bend to one side and then to the other side. Move your upper body in a circle—bend to the side, forward, to the other side, and up. Then move it in a circle the other way. Stretch out your hands, your feet, your legs, and your whole body. Shake everything out all at once. Now our bodies are wide-awake!

Modifications

This activity is designed for children who can sit and stand in a circle. To accommodate children who have movement limitations, ask them to stretch specific body parts and not necessarily all of the ones listed in the activity. For example, if a child has difficulty standing, ask him to continue to stretch while seated as you proceed through the rest of the activity.

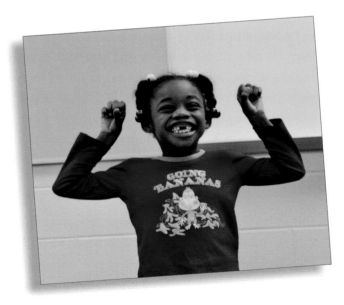

Down and Up and Down

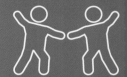

"Down and Up and Down" is a good movement game for transitioning from sitting to standing or vice versa. It's surprisingly lively for a circle activity and a great way to encourage the children to burn off excess energy so they can focus on subsequent activities.

What You Need

☼ a small space

☼ a slide whistle (optional)

What You Do

Have the children stand in a circle with plenty of room between them. Ask them to practice falling quickly, but gently, onto their seats, catching themselves with their hands. Explain that this is the safe way to do it—they should not fall hard on their seats when they go down to the floor. Use the slide whistle to signal the movement. If you do not have a slide whistle, you can sing or clap your hands. Say to the children:

Let's listen to the sound this slide whistle makes. Can you hear that it goes up and down? We are going to move our bodies along with the slide whistle. We are not only going to go up and down, we are also going to go slow and fast, along with the sound of the whistle!

I will start the whistle with a slow sound, going from up to down. Let's slowly go from standing to sitting along with the sound of the whistle. Now let's go from sitting to standing, going up as slowly as the sound of the whistle goes up. This time, I'll make the sound for going down just a little faster. I'll do it that way for standing up too. Try to move your bodies at the same speed as the whistle sound.

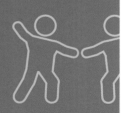

13

Continue this progression until the movement becomes very fast. Be sure to remind the children to catch themselves with their hands for this part. Finish with the children seated on the floor. Encourage them to take a few slow breaths to calm themselves after all the up-and-down movement.

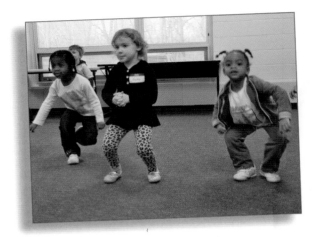

Modifications

This activity can be done with other movements based on each child's specific abilities. Children can stand in place and slowly lean their torsos from side to side, or they can turn in circles, starting slowly and increasing in speed. If they are seated, they can lift and lower their arms out in front of them, slowly at first and then more quickly. Another seated option is to have children lean their upper bodies forward and use their hands on the floor in front of them to support their upper body weight. Then have them bring their upper bodies back up to the sitting position.

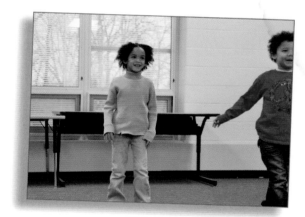

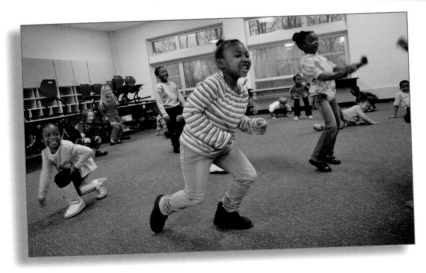

Start Fidgeting!

Teachers often want to help children get the fidgets out so they can focus on learning. "Start Fidgeting!" invites the children to fidget while they are learning! It also includes a quiet finish to help them calm down and get ready for the next part of the day.

What You Need

☼ a small space (the free dance at the end of the activity can be done moving throughout the shared space)

☼ "Shakers" instrumental (disc 2, track 36)

What You Do

Have the children sit in a circle, with plenty of space between them. Say to the children:

I see everyone has lots of energy today! Are you fidgety? We're all going to fidget together. "Fidget" means to shake and move your body. First let's fidget our heads and faces by gently shaking our heads and blinking our eyes and moving our mouths—but without talking! Now fidget just your shoulders by making small movements in many directions: up, down, forward, and back.

Try fidgeting your arms and hands. Can you fidget your whole upper body? Lifting your legs off the floor, can you fidget your legs and feet? How many parts of your body can you fidget while you are sitting in your spot? Now can you stand up while you fidget?

Let's count to ten while we fidget our whole bodies. Now freeze! Let's count to seven while we fidget. Freeze again! Let's fidget for four counts and freeze. Can you fidget for one count? Let's do that again.

Fidget. Freeze! Fidget. Freeze! Fidget. Freeze!

Now let's fidget in slow motion. Let's try to fidget our whole bodies in slow motion. Can you blink, breathe, and smile in slow motion along with the fidgeting? Now let's do the opposite: fidget as many parts of your body as you can as fast as you can!

There are other words we can use that mean the same thing as "fidget." Can you wiggle your body? Can you squirm? Can you shake? Can you jiggle?

To continue the activity, ask the children to find a home spot somewhere in the room. Say to the children:

Now we will do a fidgety, jiggly, wiggly, squirmy shake dance. You can move all around the room! Think about all the different ways we have fidgeted so far: using our different body parts, moving fast and slow, stopping and starting. I will play some music while we do our fidget dance. Play "Shakers" instrumental.

Modifications

Encourage children with movement limitations to move any parts of the body they can during the lesson. During the free dance, they can move to the music while sitting or lying down.

To end the activity, bring the children together for a quiet finish. Ask them to take a few deep breaths and wave good-bye to their fidgets.

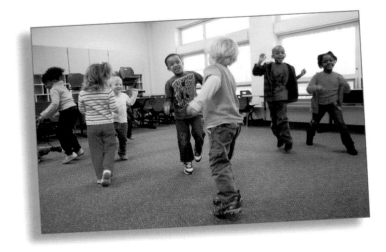

"H" Is for Hop

• • • • • • • • • • • •

"'H' Is for Hop" is a good activity for the first day of child care or preschool because it helps you and the children learn each other's names. You can repeat the activity throughout the year—the children will enjoy thinking of new movement words each time. "'H' Is for Hop" is also a counting activity and a good lead-in to the "Action Alphabet" activities in Part 4: Group Movement Explorations.

Modifications

Because the teacher will be choosing the movement performed in this activity, it can be tailored to the differing abilities of the children. For example, for a child who is blind or visually impaired, suggest an object whose sound inspires movement ideas, such as a train, a horse, a drum, or the wind.

What You Need

☼ a small space

What You Do

Begin the activity with the children standing in a circle, with enough room on each side for them to move their arms and legs. Say to the children:

Here's a fun game to help us learn each other's names! I will start. "Teacher" starts with the same sound as "tap." I will tap my foot, and then you join in. We will count out eight taps together, and then we will stop. Now who's this next to me? Mike! Let's all say, "Mike." Mike starts with the "em" sound. The word "march" starts with the same sound as "Mike." Can you march in place? Now let's all march in place six times when I say "go." Count along with me!

Continue around the circle until you have matched everyone's name with a motor skill and the children have performed it a specific number of times. If you cannot quickly come up with a motor skill for a particular letter, think of an animal name or even the name of an object. For example, "washing machine" for the letter "W" can generate the idea of moving around and around, or "xylophone" for the letter "X" can spur the idea of tapping on the imaginary instrument. Use "kangaroo" for the letter "K," and the children can perform a specific number of hops.

The next time you play "'H' Is for Hop," allow the children to come up with their own ideas for the motor skill, the animal, or the object that has the same sound as the first letter of their names.

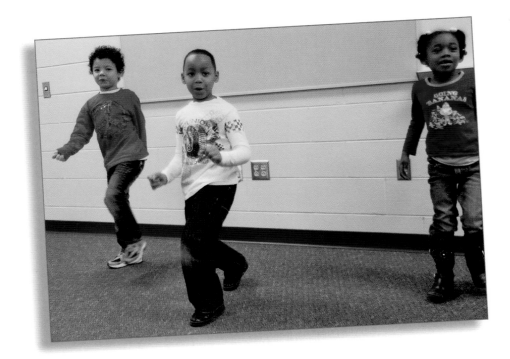

Jumpin' Jiminy

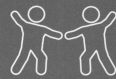

16

This is an energetic activity—great for an inside day when the children need some exercise! In addition, it introduces the correct way to perform a jump. For more jumping practice, see Activity 84: Bend and Balance, Jump and Hop.

What You Need

☼ a small space

☼ "Jumpin' Jiminy" (disc 1, track 8)

What You Do

Have the children stand in a circle with plenty of room between each other. These places will be the children's home spots. Say to the children:

> ### Modifications
>
> Children can use their arms to "jump" instead of their legs, or they can simply clap along with the rhythms. In addition, encourage them to sing with the words of the song once they have learned them.

"Jump" is a fun action word! When we jump, we use a lot of energy in the muscles of our legs and feet. Let's begin by warming up the muscles in our legs and feet so we can be ready to do some big jumps. It's important to warm up our muscles before exercising so they are ready to do big movements. Let's bend our knees slowly, and straighten them. Do it again. Let's do it slowly four times together.

Now let's bend our knees again. This time when we straighten our legs, we'll go all the way up onto our tiptoes. Bend, and straighten all the way up! Let's do that five more times together. Count with me as we do it. Can you balance on your tiptoes at the top, and hold yourself tall? If you hold your arms out to your sides, it is easier to balance.

Let's do the same thing a little faster. We will do our knee bends again, and this time, when we go up, we will go into a tiny little jump,

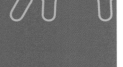

like a bounce. **Down, up, down, up—keep going! Let's do ten little bouncy jumps and bend our knees in between. Count with me. We're just like bouncing balls! We'll finish with our knees bent.**

Let's jump to some music! Play "Jumpin' Jiminy." **You can jump some more, or do whatever you wish to the lively beat in the song, but let's stay in our home spots in the circle. The song also has some slow parts when we can move slowly and rest. Follow along to the words in the song.**

We will finish with one more slow knee bend, then slowly straighten our legs again, and take a deep breath after all that jumping.

Once children are used to jumping with a good knee bend before and after each jump, the next thing to work on is a correct landing. In a correct landing, each part of the foot (toe, ball, heel) touches the floor in quick succession. Though landing in this manner is a concept that will take children a while to perform, it is important for you to be aware of how it should be done while teaching jumps.

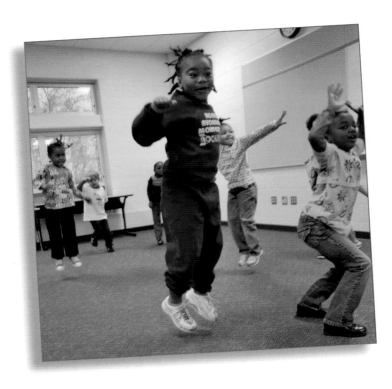

What Rhythm Is My Name?

17

"What Rhythm Is My Name?" is a fun way to create a dance. It also helps children learn to distinguish syllables in words. At the end of the exercise, you will have a rhythm dance for each person's name. Repeat it several times with the music suggested below.

What You Need

☼ a small space

☼ "All Together Now" instrumental (disc 1, track 13)

Modifications

For the child who is hearing impaired or deaf, it will be helpful for him to "see" the rhythm of each name. Use a visual aid such as a drum or tambourine to visually tap out each rhythm throughout the activity.

What You Do

Ask the children to sit on the floor in a circle. Say to them:

Let's say and clap the rhythm of each person's name. Let's begin with Samantha, and clap and say her name. It is three claps: one quiet, one loud, and one quiet. Try that with me. Now we will do this for each person as we go around the circle.

We will go around the circle again, but we will not say the person's name this time. We will just clap the rhythm of the name. After that, we'll go around once again making the rhythm of each name with our feet.

Next we will stand up, go around the circle again, make the rhythm with our feet while we are standing, and move our bodies in place while our feet make the rhythm.

Let's try that last part with music! Dance the rhythm of your own name and your classmates' names too!

Play "All Together Now" instrumental. If there is room, prompt the children to move freely about the space during this dance.

18   March with the Band

• • • • • • • • • • • • • • • •

"March with the Band" is a movement activity about the instruments that musicians play during a parade. It's a fun way to introduce different musical instruments and talk about their qualities, the ways they are played, and the sounds they make.

What You Need

☼ a small space

☼ "Marching Band" instrumental (disc 2, track 30)

☼ pictures of musical instruments

What You Do

Begin with the children seated in a circle. Say to them:

Today we're going to imagine that we're in a parade! Let's look at these pictures of musical instruments. Can you name them as I show each one? How do you think this one is played? Do you think you use your mouth to blow into it? Or do you use sticks to make a noise and beat a rhythm? Is the instrument light like the flute or heavy like the tuba? Is it large like the big bass drum or small like the little piccolo? Is it straight like the clarinet or curvy like the trombone?

Now that we've looked at all the pictures and talked about the different instruments, which one would you like to imagine you're playing? Stand up in your spot, pick up your instrument, and get ready to play. Play "Marching Band" instrumental and let the children imagine they are playing along.

First let's march in place. Can you step in time to the music? Can you turn in a small circle while you play and march? Can you turn around the other way? Now let's try a different instrument!

Let's march around our circle. Try to keep the beat with your feet, so we're all marching at the same speed. Let's turn and march around the circle the other way!

Did you try all the different instruments you wanted to play? We'll march in place one more time so you can try out some more instruments. Let's finish our game by putting all of our instruments away in my magic music bag. I will come around and you can put your instrument in the bag. That way we'll have them the next time we want to march in a parade!

Modifications

This activity can be done with the children marching in place while standing or sitting. Children can also sit while they imagine they are playing an instrument.

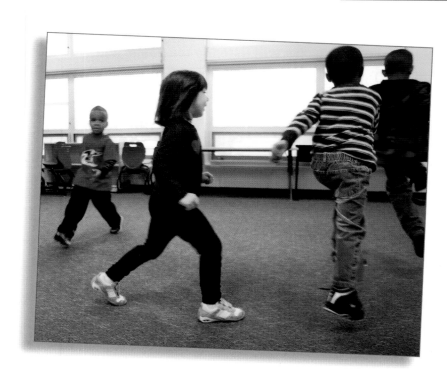

19

Big Green Alligator

A playful poem designed around the exploration of the words "up" and "down" sets the stage for the "Big Green Alligator" activity. The poem addresses additional movement opposites, such as "high" and "low" and "open" and "close."

What You Need

☼ a small space

What You Do

Have the children begin by sitting in a circle or in a home spot spread throughout the room. Say to the children:

This is a poem about an alligator who loves to ride in the elevator. He likes to go up and down. We will listen to the poem, and then we will go up and down with him! Recite the poem once all the way through to the children.

Alligator in the Elevator

A big green alligator
Jumps in the elevator
Pushing all the buttons
1, 2, 3!

Up first, then down
Up again, and down
Wait, Mr. Alligator
Wait for me!

Up, down, up, down
High, low, high, low
Open, close, open, close
Go, stop, go!

**All the way up
To the very, very top
And all the way down now
Time to stop!**

**Out we go,
Out the elevator door
See you later, alligator
No time for more!**

Recite the poem again, and after each stanza, prompt the children with the script provided below. Be sure to give the children time to complete the movement ideas. Begin by saying:

Modifications

Invite the child to help you call out the words of the poem while the others are moving. Quietly prompt her with the words before you say each line, and then have her repeat them aloud to the group with you. In addition, she can hold up a sign of a large arrow, turning it up or down each time you say those words in the poem.

Now we will dance the poem. Stand up, and let's go on the elevator with Big Green Alligator. Imagine that your home spot is an elevator. Where are the buttons to push? Where is the door?

Next read the first stanza and say to the children: **Jump into your elevator! Push the buttons 1, 2, 3!** Repeat this several times.

Read the second stanza and say to the children: **Go up onto your toes, then all the way down to the floor. Up again, and then all the way down. Now freeze!**

Read the third stanza and say to the children: **Let's go up, and let's go down** (same as in stanza 2), **and up again and down again. Let's reach high, and let's reach low. Now we'll sit down, open our arms wide, and clap them back together! Open your arms wide again, and clap them together one more time.**

Read the fourth stanza and say to the children: **In slow motion, let's go from our sitting position all the way up to standing on tiptoe with our arms reaching up. Now let's go back down to our sitting position—very, very slowly.**

Read the fifth stanza and say to the children: **Stand up, walk out of the elevator, and walk around your spot in a circle. Now walk around your spot the other way. Sit down and wave good-bye!**

20

Follow Along

. . . .

"Follow Along" is a simple activity of listening and following directions. While doing this activity, the children will learn to listen and respond to the word cues in the song.

What You Need

☼ a small space

☼ "Follow Game" (disc 1, track 4)

What You Do

Ask the children to stand in a home spot in the circle or spread throughout the shared space. Before you play the song, have the children practice the four movements suggested below while you demonstrate them. The movements do not need to be done exactly as described. Say to the children:

Let's do the shoulder shrug—Move your shoulders up and down, lifting them together or one at a time.

Now let's do the muscle mug—Pose, imagining you are a very strong bodybuilder.

Now let's do the 'squito bug—Buzz around your home spot like a mosquito.

Now let's do the wiper wug—Move your arms like windshield wipers.

Use the "Follow Game" lyrics as your movement cues. Do the "shrug," the "mug," the "bug," and the "wug" movements described above, or come up with your own!

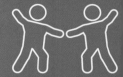

The song will begin with a short introduction inviting the children to play the Follow Game. During this musical introduction, ask the children to gently bend their knees and clap to the beat.

When the first verse begins, ask the children to do a shoulder shrug each time they hear the word "shrug."

The chorus comes next and begins with the words "And then you move," during which the children can move freely in their home spots. When they hear the word "stop," they should freeze! The next words, "For a great big hug," prompt the children to give themselves a hug. The last line in the chorus is "Now we're finished with the shoulder shrug," the prompt for the children to finish their hugs.

The second verse is the "muscle mug." The children should do a muscle mug movement each time they hear those words. Then the chorus repeats.

The third and fourth verses, the "'squito bug" and the "wiper wug," prompt the children just as the previous verses do, and the chorus repeats after each.

During the last few lines of the song, which begin with the words, "Now we're finished with the Follow Game," the children should move freely in their spots until the end of the song. At the end, ask them to freeze in a "muscle mug" shape. If there is room for the children to move around in the shared space, play the song again and allow the children to respond to the music while dancing freely.

Modifications

This activity can be performed seated. All of the movements suggested in the song can be done with the upper body.

21

Pass the Movement

• • • • • • • • • • • • • • • • • • • •

"Pass the Movement" helps children focus on the movements of other children and participate with the group. The final dance is the accumulation of all the movement ideas.

What You Need

☼ a small space

☼ "Cygnet" instrumental (disc 1, track 19)

What You Do

Have the children sit in the circle and say to them:

Do you know how to play Telephone? You play Telephone with words. You whisper a word in someone's ear, and then she passes it along by whispering the same word in the next person's ear. "Pass the Movement" is like that, except we will be passing movements instead of words! I will think of the first movement, and then one at a time, we will pass it all the way around the circle.

Modifications

If a child is blind or visually impaired, help him join in the movements by assisting him with each one. For example, with the first movement—cross your arms across your chest and then open them—hold his arms, take them across his chest, and then open them.

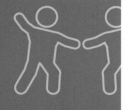

Begin with something simple, such as crossing your arms over your chest and opening them. After the movement has traveled all the way around the circle, the next person will think of a movement and pass it around. Once everyone has contributed a movement, go back and try to remember all of the movements with the children, and then do them together in sequence. Next, play the music and try to do the movements while standing. The "Pass the Movement" activity becomes a dance, because you have so many different movements to put together!

Fast and Slow, High and Low

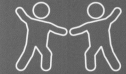

22

"Fast and Slow, High and Low" uses movement variations to teach children the concept of opposites. Teaching antonyms kinesthetically can help you introduce the concept to young children. Repeating the activity at another time can reinforce the learning. Another activity that addresses this theme is Activity 89: Opposites.

What You Need

☼ a small space, indoors or outside

☼ a drum or a tambourine

What You Do

Use a drum or a tambourine—or just clap your hands—to signal stops and starts during the activity, and to beat out the counts when you and the children count along with the movement. Ask the children to stand in a home spot in the circle. Say to them:

We're going to think about different ways of moving, which will help us learn about opposites. First let's think about the opposites "high" and "low." Can you go up on your tiptoes and reach your arms up very high? Now make yourself go as low as you can. High and low are opposites because they are very different from each other.

How about the opposites "awake" and "asleep"? While you are standing, show me your wide-awake face. Now show me your sleeping face. Go back and forth: awake, asleep, awake, asleep! They are very different faces, aren't they?

22

Now we will try the opposites "happy" and "sad" with our faces: happy, sad, happy, sad, happy! Those are very different faces and feelings too.

Let's all turn away from the center of the circle. Now let's turn back around to face the center of the circle. Let's do that a few more times: turn back, turn front, back, front, back, front. Tap the tambourine or drum, or clap your hands, to emphasize and cue the movement from "back" to "front." **"Back" and "front" are opposites, just like "high" and "low"!**

Now turn and walk away from the circle for four counts: one, two, three, four. Turn again and walk back toward your home spot. Repeat "away" for four counts, then "toward" for four counts, beating the tambourine or drum or clapping your hands as you count. Invite the children to count with you. **"Away" and "toward" are opposites!**

This time when you walk away from the circle, take little baby steps. Let's count ten little steps. Turn now and walk back toward the circle using great big giant steps. Beat the tambourine as you count, and invite the children to count with you. **Can you get back to your home spot in three big steps? Let's repeat that again. Do you see that "little" and "big" are also opposites? When you take little steps, it's a very different way to walk than when you take big steps.**

We will try the opposites "fast" and "slow" using the little steps and the big steps we just took. Turn away from the circle and take ten baby steps as fast as you can. Tap the tambourine and ask the children to count with you. **Freeze when you get to ten. Now turn around and take three slow giant steps back to the circle. Move your whole body as slowly as you can—even blink in slow motion! Can you smile in slow motion? Fast and slow are opposites too!**

The last opposites we are going to try are "loud" and "quiet." Taking four steps, can you walk away from the circle while stomping your feet? One! Two! Three! Four! Turn around now and sneak on your tiptoes as quietly as you can back to the circle! Let's do that again, and listen carefully for the difference between the opposites "loud" and "quiet."

Now let's sit down and try to remember all of the opposites we learned about today: "high" and "low," "awake" and "asleep," "happy" and "sad," "front" and "back," "toward" and "away," "little" and "big," "fast" and "slow," and "loud" and "quiet"!

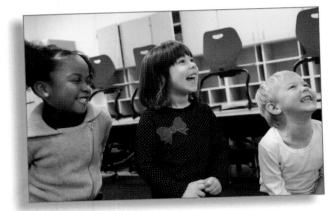

Modifications

Children can perform this activity sitting on the floor in a circle. Try these variations: the opposites "up" and "down" (lift the arms up and lower them down), "backward" and "forward" (the children can rotate on their seats), "big" and "little" (stretch tall with the body while seated, and then curl the body into a small shape). Eliminate the opposites "toward" and "away," as these require moving away from and back to the circle. Finish with "loud" and "quiet" (stomp the feet or pound the hands on the floor while sitting, and gently touch feet or pat the hands on the floor while sitting).

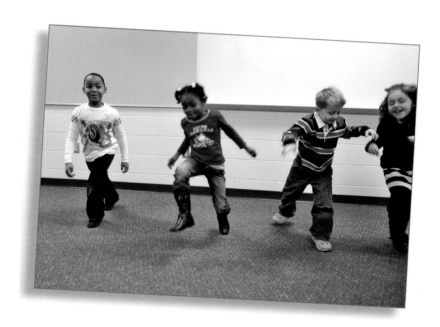

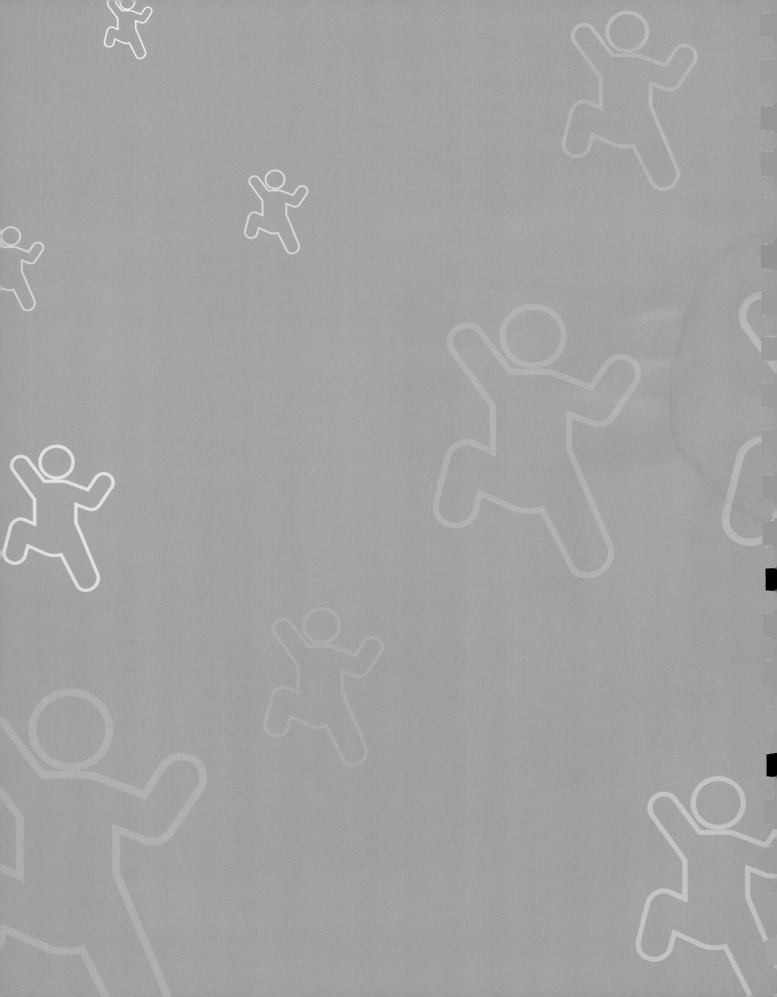

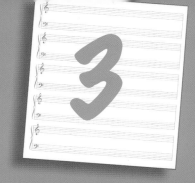

TRANSITIONS— GOING FROM HERE TO THERE

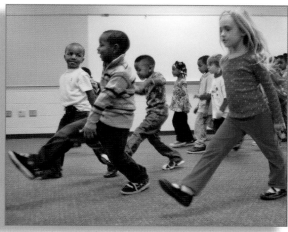

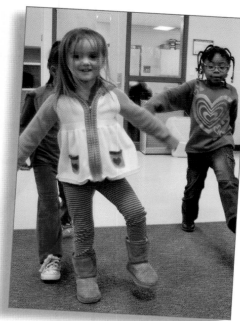

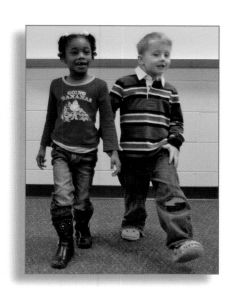

THE ACTIVITIES in "Transitions—Going from Here to There" use simple locomotor movements, or movements that travel from one place to another, to create playful transitions throughout the day. You can use the transition activities when leading the children from place to place. In addition, they are useful to help refocus the children's energy as they progress to another part of the day, such as going from a lively activity to a quieter one, in order to help ease the children into the calmer state needed to concentrate on small-motor skills and related activities. You will find a variety of movement ideas in this chapter for entering the classroom, coming to the circle, transitioning between classroom activities, and moving from outside to inside. Note that the term "starting point" refers to the place where the children begin, such as in a line or in a circle in a given area. "Destination" is the place where you want the children to be at the end of the movement activity.

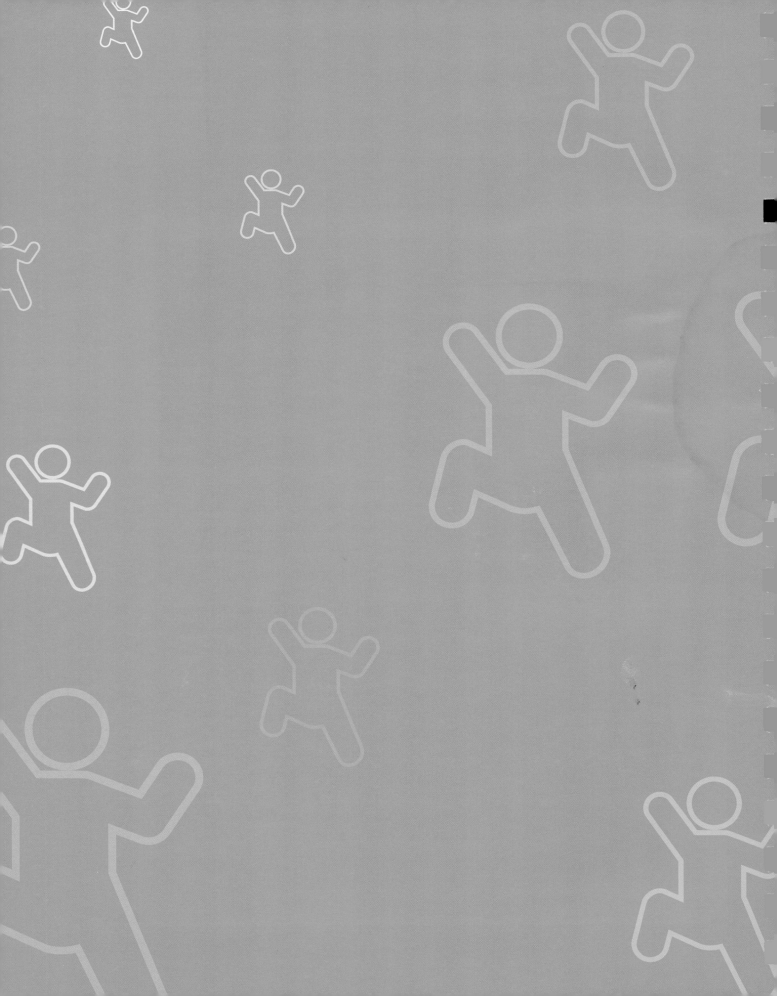

How Many Ways Can We Walk?

• • • • • • • • • • • • • •

"How Many Ways Can We Walk?" is a transition activity that can be used over several days. It is built around the simple locomotor skill of walking and uses prompts that stimulate the children's imaginations and encourage them to explore creative solutions.

What You Need

☼ a small space, indoors or outside

☼ "Dance S'More" instrumental (disc 1, track 20)

☼ a portable drum or a small sign with green on one side and red on the other (optional)

What You Do

Line up the children at the starting point: for instance, in the hallway, outside, or at the classroom door. Point out the destination. You can say, "We will all be walking from here, our starting point, down this hallway to the door of the classroom, our destination." Establish a movement cue such as a hand clap, a beat on a portable drum, or the flash of a small sign showing green (for go) on one side and red (for stop) on the other. Say to the children:

Today we will do an activity about walking! I want you to think about how you can change the way you step. As you go toward the classroom, make a change in your walk so that it looks and feels different than it usually does, but make sure it's still a walk!

23

I will clap my hands one time (or beat the drum or hold up the green sign), **and that will be your signal to walk. Each of you will do this in the order you are lined up, and you will finish in the same order in the line when we get to the classroom** (or other destination). **Here comes my signal, so let's go!**

The first child will begin, and if he doesn't change his walk, give him one of the following movement cues:

- **Can you take bigger steps than you usually do?**

- **Can you walk very slowly?**

- **Can you lift one leg higher?**

- **Can you walk sideways?**

- **Can you lift your arms high in the air while you walk?**

Once the children have caught on and are able to come up with new ideas, say:

Look at all the different kinds of walking! Did you know there were so many ways to walk? Now that we're all lined up in the room (or at the end of the hallway) **and you are still in your line, can you do your walk without traveling? Try to keep doing your new walk, but do it in place. I'll clap my hands again** (or beat the drum or hold up the stop sign). **When I do, I want everyone to freeze in the middle of a step from your new way of walking. That will signal the end of our game!**

Continue this transition activity for the next several days. Consider narrowing the children's choices by focusing each day's activity using the elements of dance in different ways. For example:

- tempo variations: the children can walk in slow or fast motion; walk in a choppy rhythm; walk for four steps and freeze, and then repeat.

- energy variations: the children can walk heavily as an elephant; walk light as a feather; walk as though trudging through goopy mud; walk as though moving through water; walk stiff as a robot; walk as if sad or happy.

- body-part variations: the children can walk with one or both knees high; move their arms in new ways—for example, swinging them energetically or holding them in a specific shape; lead their walk with a body part, such as an elbow, shoulder, or head; make funny faces; make a twisty shape with their bodies as they walk.

- spatial variations: the children can walk in a curlicue pattern; walk high or low; walk backward or sideways; walk with baby steps or giant steps; take one large step and then one tiny step, and then repeat the pattern.

A nice musical accompaniment for this activity is "Dance S'More" instrumental. The musical accompaniment is optional, but it provides a lively background for the walks. If you decide to use music with this activity, start it once the children are lined up and ready. While using the music, you will still find it helpful to use a sound or sign to cue the children to begin and end their walking patterns.

Modifications

If the children are not readily coming up with their own ideas, keep in mind each child's abilities as you give movement suggestions. For example, if a child is not able to balance well, suggest that she take small steps for her walking variation and encourage her to place her arms out to the side to help her balance.

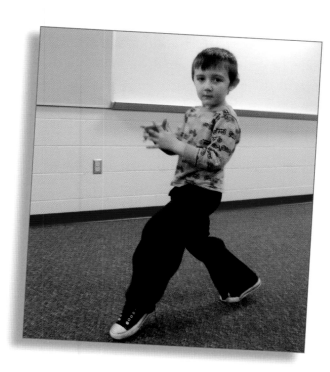

24

Space Suits

• • • • • • • • • • •

"Space Suits" is a transition activity that helps children begin to understand the idea of moving together in a shared space. It also helps introduce them to the concept that everyone's personal space should be respected—an important classroom management tool for all movement activities. Activity 75: Grocery Space Trip is a good follow-up.

What You Need

☼ a small space, indoors or outside (the free movement at the end of the activity can be done moving throughout the shared space)

☼ a picture of an astronaut in a space suit (optional)

What You Do

Line up the children at the starting point of the transition activity: for instance, in the hallway, outside, or at the classroom door. Point out the destination. You can say, "We will all be walking from here, our starting point, down this hallway to the door of the classroom, our destination." Say to the children:

Today we're going to enter the classroom in a very special way. We're going to put on imaginary suits—just like astronauts wear! Show the children a picture of an astronaut's suit. **These suits create a big bubble around the astronauts and protect them while they are in outer space.**

Let's slip into our astronaut suits and fasten them carefully. Now let's pull on our special boots, one on each foot. Finally, let's put on our big astronaut helmets. Imagine the big suit all around you. Can you feel it? Do you see how the space suits are like a bubble around each person?

We're ready to go into outer space! Let's prepare for takeoff by crouching down low, as if we were rockets ready to launch, and

counting backward together from ten: ten, nine, eight, seven, six, five, four, three, two, one! Our rocket ship is taking off! Jump as high as you can into the air! Now let's imagine we are flying above Earth. Look at the moon and the other planets!

Let's go out of our rocket ship and do a space walk! We will walk to the classroom, being careful not to bump into anyone else's space suit. We're floating in outer space! What do we see around us?

The children should continue moving this way until they arrive at the transitional activity destination. If you want to end the activity at this point, prompt the children to climb back in the rocket ship and fly back to Earth. Continue with the activity if your room or outside area can accommodate the children moving freely about.

Modifications

A child who is in a wheelchair can participate in this activity with a little reminder to all before the activity begins. If he can operate his wheelchair himself, ask him and the other children to imagine a space suit big enough to go around the whole chair and to think about that as he moves with the others. Remind him to maneuver slowly and carefully through the shared space. If someone is pushing him, remind everyone that the imaginary space suit will be big enough to include that person as well.

Now let's walk all around the room in our space suits. While we are walking, let's practice staying far enough away from each other so that every astronaut has lots of room. Don't let your space suit touch anyone else's space suit.

It's time to get back in our rocket ship and fly back to Earth. Hold on! Our rocket ship has landed. Climb out! Let's take off our suits and hang them up. That way we'll know where they are when we want to use them again.

The lesson in this transition activity—to develop the awareness of personal space (one's own as well as that of others)—can be applied throughout the day whenever children are moving freely together during movement sessions and other group activities. Repeating the reminder "Like an astronaut's suit, remember the space around you and the other children" can help reinforce being cognizant and respectful of the others with whom they are moving in the shared space.

If at first the children do not grasp the concept of the space suit, here is a suggestion for approaching the activity. Explain that their space suits are as wide across as their arms when they hold their arms straight out at their sides. Proceed through the activity, and when the children finish putting on their imaginary suits, ask them to hold their arms out throughout the entire activity until they take off their imaginary suits. If they do this successfully, repeat the activity and ask them to imagine they still have their arms open wide. This will help them maintain the same distance between each other as they move about.

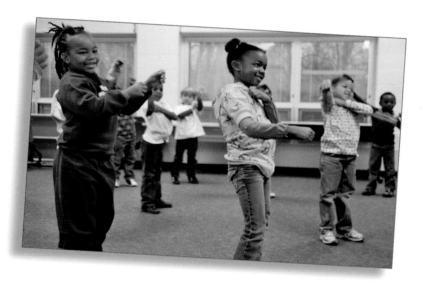

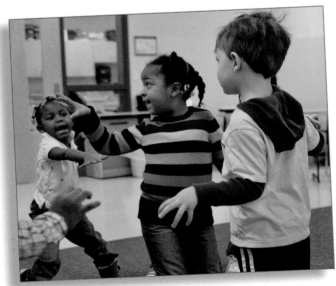

How Do Animals Move?

"How Do Animals Move?" is a transition activity that can be used over several days. The movement ideas are generated from the various ways animals move, as well as the unique qualities of different animals. The specific animals are based on the preferences of each child, within parameters chosen by the teacher.

What You Need

☼ a small space

☼ "Zoo Babies" instrumental (disc 2, track 42)

☼ a portable drum or a small sign with green on one side and red on the other (optional)

What You Do

Line up the children at the starting point of the transition activity: for instance, in the hallway, outside, or at the classroom door. Point out the destination. You can say, "We will all be walking from here, our starting point, down this hallway to the door of the classroom, our destination." Establish a movement cue such as a hand clap, a beat on a portable drum, or the flash of a small sign showing green (for go) on one side and red (for stop) on the other. Say to the children:

Today we're going to think about how different animals move. Think of your favorite animal. One by one, I'm going to ask you what that animal is. I'm also going to ask you to move like that animal as you make your way to the door (or to wherever their destination is).

I will clap my hands one time (or beat the drum or hold up the green sign), **and that will be your signal to walk. Each of you will do this, one by one,**

in the order you are lined up. When I clap my hands again, which means it is time for you to stop, turn and watch the other children as they move like animals. Here comes my signal, so let's go!

Look at all the different kinds of animals! Enough to fill a zoo! The children can form a loose line as they gather to watch others.

Now that we've all arrived at the door, I'll clap my hands again (or beat the drum or hold up the stop sign). **When I do, I want each of you to freeze in the shape of your favorite animal. That will signal the end of our game!**

Continue this transition activity for the next several days. Consider narrowing the children's choices by focusing each day's activity in different ways. For example:

- animals that fly
- animals that swim
- animals that live in cold places
- animals that are found on a farm

Modifications

You can ask a child being pushed in her wheelchair to use her arms, head, and hands to move like the animal. For example, if she chooses a whale for her animal, encourage her to toss her head as if she is moving in the ocean and coming up for air, and to use her arms and hands as fins.

A nice musical accompaniment for this activity is "Zoo Babies" instrumental. The musical accompaniment is optional, but it provides an upbeat tempo for the walks. If you decide to use music with this activity, start it once the children are ready to begin their animal movements. To finish the activity, ask the children to freeze in their favorite animal shape when you stop the music.

Tightrope Walker

26

"Tightrope Walker," which can be done indoors or outside, helps children practice body control, focus, and balance as they move from one place to another.

What You Need

☼ a small space, indoors or outside

☼ masking tape, string or yarn, or chalk; a portable drum or a small sign with green on one side and red on the other (optional); a picture of a tightrope walker (optional)

What You Do

To create a tightrope—a straight line—for the children to walk on, use masking tape on an uncovered floor or string or yarn on a rug. Hold one end of the string or yarn and tie the other end to the leg of a desk or chair. Use chalk if you do this activity outdoors. The tightrope should be six to eight feet long. Challenge the children to walk a longer tightrope if you repeat the activity. Line up the children at the starting point: for instance, in the hallway, outside, or at the classroom door. Point out the destination. You can say, "We will all be walking from here, our starting point, down this hallway to the door of the classroom, our destination." Show the children a picture of someone walking a tightrope. Say to the children:

Have you ever seen a picture of a tightrope walker or visited the circus and seen a tightrope walker in person? Tightrope walkers have to have very good balance, don't they? We're going to imagine we're walking on a very high and very narrow tightrope, which is this line of masking tape (or string or yarn). **Keep your eyes on your feet as you step on the tightrope. Try to place your whole foot on the rope when you take a step, and then change to the other foot very carefully. Don't try to go fast—it's important**

to take your time so you'll stay on the rope! Hold your arms out wide at your sides to help you keep your balance.

I will clap my hands one time (or beat the drum or hold up the green sign) **to let each of you know when to climb high up the imaginary ladder and start across the tightrope. When you get all the way to the end of the tightrope, imagine you are climbing down the long ladder back to the ground. Then sit down and watch the other tightrope walkers come across.**

Start the children one by one. Make sure a child is at least halfway across the tightrope before you cue the next child to begin.

Modifications

A wider path can be designated for those children who are unable to balance well or walk the narrow tightrope. The wider path can be the whole space between two straight rows of blocks, or between two lines of tape, string, yarn, or chalk. The path can be much shorter for children who are not able to sustain the activity for more than a few steps.

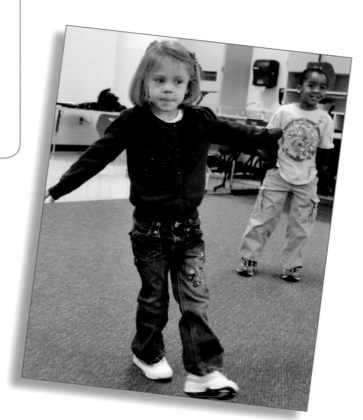

Surprise!

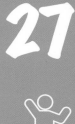

"Surprise!" is a great activity for transitions from one place to another or from one part of the daily routine to another. It's filled with a variety of movement prompts that help get children's creative juices flowing!

What You Need

☼ a small space, indoors or outside

☼ three-by-five-inch index cards (one for each child)

What You Do

Before you begin the activity, write a different movement idea on each index card. Choose from any of the ideas below, and add any that you know the children would enjoy:

- walk sideways

- take baby steps

- take giant steps

- walk in a zigzag pattern

- hop

- jump

- walk as low as you can

- walk as high as you can

- march, lifting your knees up high and swinging your arms

- walk as if you are carrying a huge bag of rocks on your back

- float like a balloon, and then pop when you get into the room

- sneak into the room silently

- make a funny face while you march

- walk in a curlicue pattern

- make a funny shape with your body before you start walking and a different one when you are in the room

- clap your hands over your head while you march

- do traveling jumping jacks

- stomp as though walking through mud puddles

- walk sideways on your tiptoes

- hop while you clap your hands

- alternate steps and jumps (for example, three steps and one jump) and repeat the pattern

- slide as though ice-skating

Modifications

Because you will be choosing and writing specific movement prompts ahead of time, prepare the ideas based on the differing abilities of the children. If you know the instructions for this exercise will be difficult for a specific child, choose something simple and straightforward, such as "take baby steps," and then do the movement with her. When she catches on, encourage her to continue the movement to the destination by herself.

Line up the children at the starting point: for example, in the hallway, outside, or at the classroom door. Point out the destination. You can say, "We will all be walking from here, our starting point, down this hallway to the door of the classroom, our destination." Say to the children:

Today we are each going to enter the classroom in a different way. I am going to choose a movement for each of you from one of these cards. Then one by one, you will do that movement as you enter the room.

If the destination is a small area, ask the children to sit down once they have reached the destination and watch others as they move in various ways. If the destination is a large space, allow the children to continue their movements once they reach the destination. Provide a cue, such as a hand clap, once everyone has reached the destination. Ask them to freeze for four counts and then go down to the floor for four counts to finish in a seated position. If there is time, use the cards again to assign different movements, or ask the children to try some of the movements they saw the other children doing.

Try repeating this activity another day, guiding the children to create their own ways of moving. "Surprise!" can also be done in a larger space, outside or inside, and not as a transition from one place to another but with the children moving freely in response to the movement prompts. If you want all the children to try each movement prompt together, hold the cards up one by one while all of the children respond to each one.

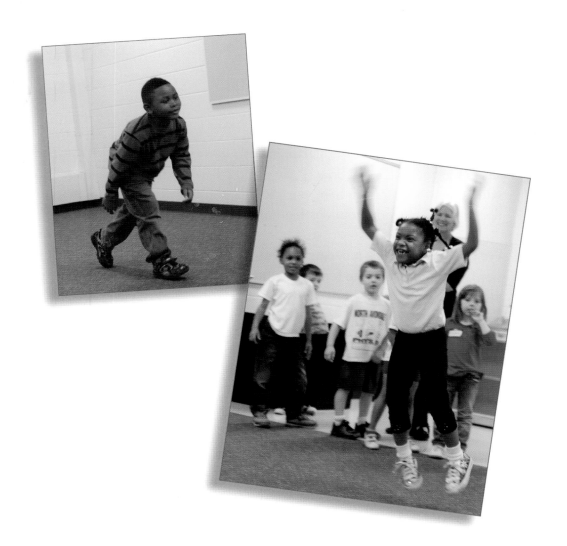

28

Follow My Footsteps

Prompts about different movement qualities, such as imagining what it is like to move through mud or snow, are used to encourage children to try new ways of moving as they follow you from a starting point to a destination.

What You Need

☼ a small space, indoors or outside

What You Do

Line up the children at the starting point: for instance, in the hallway, outside, or at the classroom door. Point out the destination. You can say, "We will all be walking from here, our starting point, down this hallway to the door of the classroom, our destination." Say to the children:

We're going to play a movement game to go back inside (or other destination). **I'm going to be the leader, so line up behind me as we get ready to start.**

Have you ever seen the footprints you make with your boots when you walk in the mud or snow, or the footprints you make when you walk barefoot in the wet sand? We're going to pretend that we can make footprints while we're walking. Try to follow my exact steps by imagining they are footprints.

While the children are following you, prompt their imaginations by suggesting these ideas:

- Let's imagine we're in the mud. I have to pull hard to get my boots out of the squishy mud!

- Now the mud isn't so squishy, and there are lots of puddles. Let's stomp in the puddles! Look how much we're splashing!

- Now we're in the snow. It's slushy—slide your boots through the slush.

- Let's imagine now that we're in very deep snow. Can you lift your legs very high each time you take a step?

- Uh-oh, it's getting icy! Let's slide on the ice, but be careful not to slip!

- It's finally warm now, and we're at the beach. Our bare feet will make footprints in the sand, just like our boots did in the snow. Follow me as we walk through the sand toward the ocean. Do you feel the warm sand on your feet? Look at the patterns our feet are making in the sand. Let's splash through the waves as they wash up on the shore!

Depending on how much time and space you have for the transition, allow the children to explore each new idea. If the children continue to be engaged, "Follow My Footsteps" can grow from a transitional activity into a longer movement study. The children can contribute their own ideas and explore and expand the various movement prompts.

Modifications

If you have a child who uses a wheelchair, place him in front of you so you can push him while you lead the other children. Ask him to use his hands in the air as if they were his feet, imagining them in the mud, snow, and sand during the prompts. The other children can follow along behind you.

29

Quiet As a Mouse

The image of sneaking and trying to move as silently as possible can help children stay focused and quiet during transitions.

What You Need

☼ a small space, indoors or outside

What You Do

Line up the children at the starting point: in the hallway, outside, or at the classroom door. Or remain seated if the children have just completed a seated activity, such as circle time, as in the example below. Point out the destination. You can say, "We will all be walking from here, our starting point, down this hallway to the door of the classroom, our destination." Say to the children:

We're going to move from our sitting positions in the circle to standing in a line by the door across the room (or other destination). **Before we start, let's think of some things that move quietly. How about a cat? A mouse? What else moves around without making any noise?**

Stand up as quietly as you can, staying in your spot in the circle. How do you walk when you don't want anyone to hear you? Do you tiptoe? When you talk, do you whisper? Let's all put our index fingers to our mouths and whisper, "Shhhhh!"

Now we're going to see how quietly we can move. I'll go around the circle and gently tap you when it's your turn to move. Like a cat or a mouse, touch your feet silently on the floor each time you take a step. As we arrive at

Modifications

If a child is blind or visually impaired, ask another child or an aide to hold her hand during the transition, and help her find her place in the line at the destination.

the door one by one, let's make our line by the door nice and straight. Remember, we don't want anyone to hear us—not one sound!

Okay, we all moved without making any noise, and we ended up in a nice straight line by the door! You were all as quiet as mice!

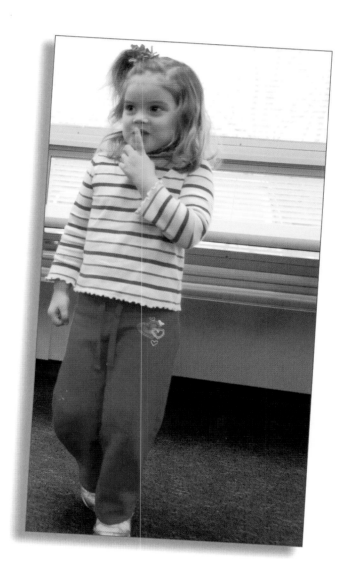

30

Stepping-Stones

Movement prompts can generate individual responses as well as solutions developed through group participation. "Stepping-Stones" does both: each of the children contributes ideas to create an imaginary outdoor walk, which the group then explores together.

What You Need

☼ a small space

What You Do

Loosely cluster the children in a group at the starting point: for instance, in the hallway, outside, or at the classroom door. Point out the destination. You can say, "We will all be walking from here, our starting point, down this hallway to the door of the classroom, our destination." Be sure to allow children time to develop movement ideas after each prompt. As you see them respond with new ideas, mention these to the group. "Look, Maya is jumping over the sprinkler. Let's all try that!" Encourage them to try other children's creative solutions. Say to the children:

Let's imagine we're taking a walk outside. Let's go together! We'll open the door (gesture as if you are opening a door and ask the children to open a door too) **and walk down the steps. Watch out, there's a sprinkler on the lawn. Dodge it—or go through it!**

Now let's go down the hill toward the woods. What do you think we'll see in the woods?

Finally, we're in the woods. I see a beautiful brook rushing by. We'll need to cross it. What should we do? Should we hop on the stepping-

stones, walk over the little bridge, or hold hands and step carefully through the water? Let's try crossing the brook all three ways. Here we go!

Look! A big hill! Let's climb all the way up. Isn't it hard to climb such a steep slope? What can we see from the top?

It's time to get back home. Let's head back down the hill and take a shortcut through those tall bushes. We can't see over the top of them. I wonder what's on the other side? Let's try to move the leaves aside as we slowly make our way through the thick bushes and step high over all the roots. What do you see now that we've made it through?

At last we arrive home. Let's sit down and talk about our walk. What was your favorite part? Why?

Modifications

If it's not possible for a child to do the movements mentioned in this story, simply create your own story. Your imaginary outing can be a train trip, and the children can sit in a line or a circle and respond with what they "see" out the train's window. Incorporate the movement into the train's "turning" ("Let's lean this way!") and the ups and downs in the track ("Did you feel us go over that big bump?").

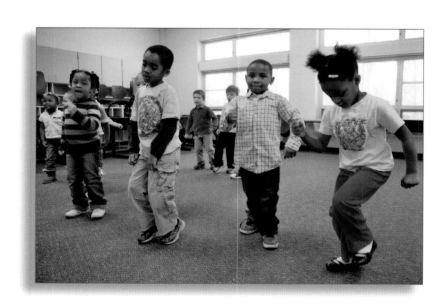

31

Cars, Cars, Cars!

. . . .

"Cars, Cars, Cars!" can be a quick transitional activity, or it can be developed into a longer movement activity with children moving about a larger space in their imaginary cars.

What You Need

☼ a small space

☼ "Savannah" instrumental (disc 2, track 35)

☼ three circles, six inches in diameter, one each cut from red, yellow, and green construction paper

What You Do

Line up the children at the starting point: for instance, in the hallway, outside, or at the classroom door. Point out the destination. You can say, "We will all be walking from here, our starting point, down this hallway to the door of the classroom, our destination." Play "Savannah" instrumental as you begin this activity. Say to the children:

Do you like to ride in the car? What's your favorite color car? Is your car big or small? Now why don't you get in your car, fasten your seat belt, and start your engine. Let's imagine we're driving our own cars!

We'll put our cars in a line, and I will give you each the green light when it's your turn to go. All right! Let's imagine this hallway (or other location) **back to the classroom is our road.**

Modifications

For a child who is hearing impaired or deaf, make sure to use the visual traffic signals so that he knows when to stop and start throughout the activity. If a child is visually impaired or blind, pair him with another child or an aide and supplement the signs with clear verbal explanations: "I am holding up the green sign. That means go! Now I am holding up the yellow sign. Slow down!"

Stay in line as you drive your car, just like you see drivers doing when you ride in an adult's car.

Let's all try to drive at the same speed. We'll drive very carefully and watch out for all the other cars. Look, here's a traffic light. Walk along at the front of the line of cars and hold up a green, yellow, or red paper traffic light as needed. **It's changing from green to yellow, so we'll put on our brakes to slow down. It's red now, so let's come to a complete stop! We have to wait until it turns green to go. Okay, it's green again. Let's drive!**

Continue the driving until the children have reached the destination. To bring the transition activity to a close, ask the children to park their cars, turn off the engines, take off their seat belts, and get out of their cars.

32

Conga Line

• • • • • • • • • • •

"Conga Line" is a fun, upbeat movement transition activity. The children learn the conga rhythm with clapping, then respond to this beat with a variety of movements. This activity can be done inside or outdoors, with or without music.

What You Need

☼ a small space

☼ "Shakers" instrumental (disc 2, track 36)

What You Do

Begin this transition activity with the children seated in a circle. Point out the destination. For example, you can say, "We will all be walking from here, our starting point, down this hallway to the door of the classroom, our destination." Say to the children:

We're going to learn a rhythm called the conga. It has four beats. Clap four times with me: one, two, three, four. This time, we're going to make the fourth beat strong, which is called an accent. One, two, three, FOUR! One, two, three, FOUR! This "one-two-three-FOUR" rhythm is the conga rhythm.

Try it with your feet while sitting. Can you move your feet to the rhythm and clap it too? Now stand in place and try the rhythm with your feet: step one, step two, step three, strong-step FOUR. Repeat this with the children several times. Encourage them to count the rhythm out loud with you while they step in place to the beat.

Now, on the strong fourth beat, instead of stepping down onto your foot, stretch your leg to the side and touch your toes to the floor. Still standing in place, try putting it all together: step one, step two, step

three, touch-floor-with-toes four. **Step one, step two, step three, touch-floor-with-toes four. This step-step-step-touch movement is the conga dance!**

Let's try the conga dance standing together in a line. I'll be the leader. I'll place you in a line behind me so there's space between each person. Let's start out very slowly. We'll step forward on one, two, and three, and then we'll touch our toes to the side on four. Now we'll try it again, a little faster this time. Walk one, two, three, touch four. Walk one, two, three, touch four. Good!

Now let's try it again, clapping our hands on that strong fourth beat, at the same time we touch our toes to the side. Can we try it a little faster? Now we'll do our conga dance to music! Play "Shakers" instrumental.

Lead the children away from the starting point while they are doing the conga dance to music. As you approach the destination, turn off the music and recreate the conga beat with your voice; indicate that you are coming to the end of the activity and say to the children:

One, two, slow, DOWN, one, two, slow, DOWN, one, two, and, STOP!

Teaching children the conga rhythm before the dance helps them transfer it into their bodies as they step to the beat of the music. Don't be concerned at first about which foot takes the first step and which foot (toes) touches the floor to the side. As the children become comfortable with the conga dance, you can begin demonstrating the concepts of "right" and "left." Point to your right leg (or tap it, and have the children do the same to their own right legs) and say to the children:

We'll start on the right foot. We step right, left, right, and then we touch our left toes to the floor! Now we do the same thing starting on our left foot.

By following your dancing, the children can begin to understand kinesthetically the concepts of "right" and "left."

Modifications

A child who is blind or visually impaired can participate in this activity. Once she and the other children have learned the beat and the movements, first by clapping, then stepping in place, let her stand in front of you while you put your hands on her shoulders. (The other children will be lined up behind you.) Gently guide her as she begins to move so you can control her direction and pace.

32

[91]

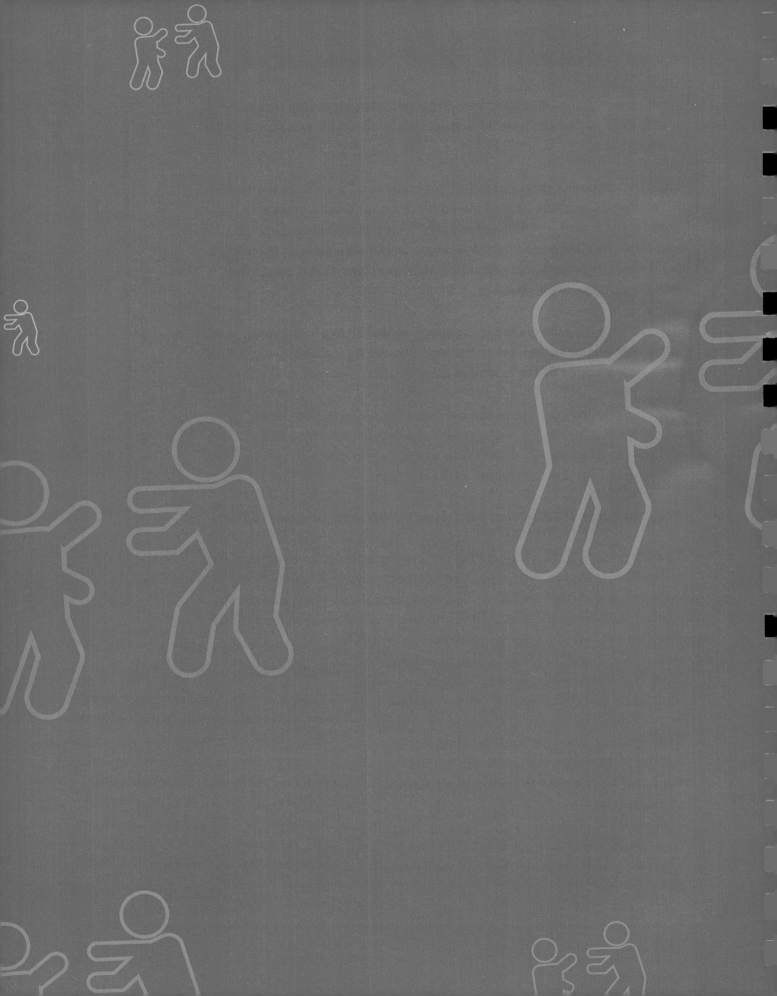

GROUP MOVEMENT EXPLORATIONS

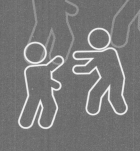

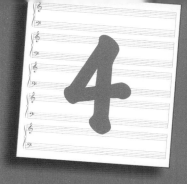

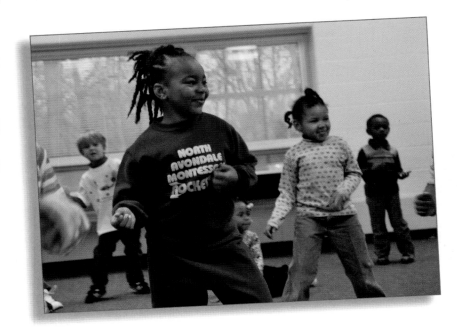

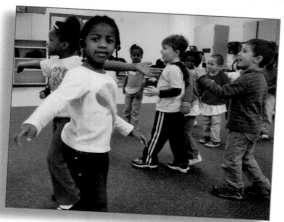

EDUCATORS HAVE IDENTIFIED skills, concepts, and benchmarks important to the development of the growing child. These early childhood standards, which may vary from state to state, fall into four major categories: English language arts, mathematics, social studies, and science. Activities in "Group Movement Explorations" span the spectrum of these categories, addressing and playfully exploring many important early childhood academic concepts. The group movement activities can be used as part of a themed lesson or as an independent movement study, and each one includes many opportunities for creative exploration. The activities are organized in the following manner:

- language and literacy (activities 33 through 55)—movement that explores concepts such as vocabulary acquisition, phonemic awareness, early reading, and letter recognition

- numbers, shapes, and patterns (activities 56 through 63)—movement that explores concepts such as numbers and counting, spatial sense, and patterns

- science (activities 64 through 72)—movement that explores concepts such as Earth and space, life science, physical science, and energy and motion

- social studies (activities 73 through 77)—movement that addresses concepts such as history, daily life, cultures, and geography

Action Alphabet "A"

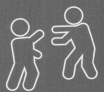

Each "Action Alphabet" activity is an independent and fun letter exploration with a short script for the teacher. An "Action Alphabet" activity can be used in conjunction with letter studies or as a simple movement and shape activity.

What You Need

☼ a small space

☼ a large card showing the capital letter "A"

Explores language and literacy!

What You Do

Begin the letter exploration with each of the children standing in a home spot in a circle, with plenty of room between each child. During the activity, have the children return to their home spots whenever necessary. Hold up a large card showing the capital letter "A." Say to the children:

The letter "A" sounds just like its name! It's the first letter of the alphabet. Do you see that the letter "A" is made from three straight lines? We have straight lines in our bodies. Can you make your whole body into a straight line? How about just your arms? Can you hold them out straight? Now let's try your legs. Can you lift one leg, put it down, then the other, keeping them straight the whole time?

Let's make straight lines with our bodies on the floor. Be careful not to bump into your neighbor! Lying on your back, can you make a straight line with one leg lifted into the air? Put that one down and try the other. Now bring both legs up at once, and see the big straight line they make together. Can you move your feet apart, and see the shape of the two slanted straight lines your legs make in the air? Bring your feet back together to make one big straight line. Let's do that several times: open, close, open, close.

33

Do the same thing with your arms. First bring one arm up in the air, then the other, and bring your hands together. Then open your arms to make two slanted lines, and bring them back together. Repeat the movement: open, close, open, close.

Now stretch your whole body into one long line on the floor. Let's open and close our arms and legs at the same time: open, close, open, close. Now roll over so you're face down, and push yourself up to your hands and feet, with your seat high in the air. Do you see that in this position you're like an upside-down triangle, with two slanted lines? Walk your hands back to your feet—one, two, three, four—and slowly uncurl your body until you are standing up in a straight line again!

Modifications

Prompt children who have difficulty making shapes with their whole bodies to use body parts instead. You can, for example, encourage a child to try making a straight line with his arm, hand, or fingers.

You can ask the child to identify and hold up a picture of a straight line while the other children make the same shape with their bodies. She can hold up the letter card for you and point to different parts of the letter while you instruct the other children to make the shapes. For instance, the child can point to a slanted line while you prompt the others to make their bodies into a slanted line; this helps her develop letter recognition and be an active participant in the group.

Give the child an opportunity to call out some of the prompts in the lesson. The child can help you call out "open" or "close."

Let's make the long straight line of our body into a slanted line. Slanted lines are straight, but instead of going up and down, they look and feel like they're tilted. Let's tilt and sway from side to side, keeping our bodies straight, but now, look how we're slanted when we rock from side to side!

To finish the activity, let's hold an imaginary crayon. Look at the letter "A" one more time. It has two slanted lines. Can you make a line in the air that slants from here to here, then, starting at the top again, join another line to it that slants from here to here? Next make a line that crosses these two through the middle. You made the letter "A" in the air! Try it again!

Remember that the kinesthetic exploration of letters is what is important, not the finished product. Whether or not he accomplishes the exact letter shape, it is the child's attempts to make the shapes with his body that is the valuable learning experience.

Action Alphabet "B"

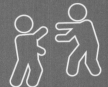

Each "Action Alphabet" activity is an independent and fun letter exploration with a short script for the teacher. An "Action Alphabet" activity can be used in conjunction with letter studies or as a simple movement and shape activity.

What You Need

Explores language and literacy!

☼ a small space

☼ a large card showing the capital letter "B"

What You Do

Begin the letter exploration with each of the children standing in a home spot in a circle, with plenty of room between each child. During the activity, have the children return to their home spots whenever necessary. Hold up a large card showing a capital letter "B." Say to the children:

Every letter in the alphabet is made up of shapes. The letter "B" contains one straight line. Will you make yourself into a straight line? You can see that the letter "B" has curved shapes in it too. Can you find some curved shapes in your body? Can you make curves with your arms? Legs? Can you make your whole body into a curve?

Let's play a game that will help us feel the difference between curved and straight. When I clap my hands, I will say either "curve" or "straight." You will make that shape with different parts of your body, or with your whole body, and hold it until I clap my hands again. Be careful not to bump into your neighbor.

Now I'm going to give you three instructions in a row, more quickly than before. Are you ready? Straight, curve, curve! The children should do one

34

straight and then two different curved shapes. **There you go! That is the letter "B"—straight, curve, curve!**

Now look at the "B" one more time. Can you try to make the whole letter "B" with your body? Can you try it lying on the floor? Try it standing one more time. Look at all those straight and curved lines!

Modifications

Prompt children who have difficulty making shapes with their whole bodies to use body parts instead. You can, for example, encourage a child to try making a curved shape with his arm, hand, or fingers.

You can ask the child to identify and hold up a picture of a straight or curved line while the other children make the same shape in their bodies. He can hold up the letter card for you and point to different parts of the letter while you instruct the other children to make the shapes. For instance, the child can point to a curve while you prompt the others to make their bodies into a curved shape; this can help him develop letter recognition and be an active participant in the group.

Give the child an opportunity to call out some of the prompts in the lesson. The child can help you call out "curve" or "straight."

Remember that the kinesthetic exploration of letters is what is important, not the finished product. Whether or not she accomplishes the exact letter shape, it is the child's attempts to make the shapes with her body that is the valuable learning experience.

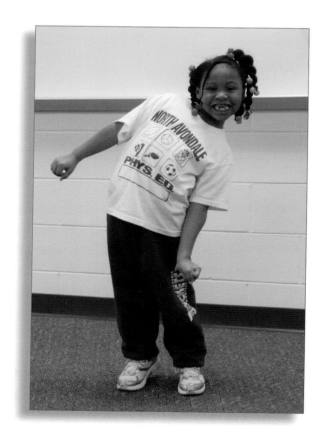

Action Alphabet "C"

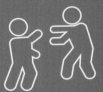

Each "Action Alphabet" activity is an independent and fun letter exploration with a short script for the teacher. An "Action Alphabet" activity can be used in conjunction with letter studies or as a simple movement and shape activity.

What You Need

- ☼ a small space

- ☼ a large card showing the capital letter "C"

Explores language and literacy!

What You Do

Begin the letter exploration with each of the children standing in a home spot in a circle, with plenty of room between each child. During the activity, have the children return to their home spots whenever necessary. Hold up a large card showing a capital letter "C." Say to the children:

Let's explore the letter "C." It's a big curve! We can make our whole bodies into a curve, just like the letter "C." Can you bend to the side while you hold your arms close to your body? If you bend your knees a little and hold your arms over your head, you can make yourself into an even bigger curve. Can you hold your curved "C" shape while you turn around?

Bring your arms down, and try making the "C" shape by bending to the other side, first with your arms down, and then bending your knees and holding your arms over your head to make a bigger curve. Turn around while you are bending this way too. Can you jump while holding your "C" shape? Can you hop on one leg and still hold your curved shape?

35

Now let's make a "C" shape by bending another way. Bend forward from your waist while your arms are next to your sides, and you're making another "C" shape! Can you reach all the way to the floor and support yourself on your feet and hands? Feel your back making a curve. Your body is making another great big "C" shape! Bend your knees, touch them to the floor, and slowly lower yourself all the way to the floor.

Let's make our bodies into a "C" shape while lying on the floor. First try it on your side, then roll over and try it on your other side.

Now try one more "C" shape. While sitting, lift your legs into the air, so that only your seat is touching the floor. Can you hold this shape and balance in it? Do you see the big curved shape your body is making?

Modifications

Prompt children who have difficulty making shapes with their whole bodies to use body parts instead. You can, for example, encourage a child to try making a curved shape with her arm, hand, or fingers.

You can ask the child to identify and hold up a picture of a curved line while the other children make the same shape with their bodies. She can hold up the letter card for you and point to different parts of the letter while you instruct the other children to make the shapes. For instance, the child can point to a curve while you prompt the others to make their bodies into a curved shape; this will help her develop letter recognition and be an active participant in the group.

Let's finish our game by trying to remember all of the different ways we made "C" shapes with our bodies, and do each of them one more time. Who can remember a standing "C" shape? Try it again! What about one we made by leaning forward? Lying down? Sitting? What's your favorite way to make a "C" shape?

Remember that the kinesthetic exploration of letters is what is important, not the finished product. Whether or not he accomplishes the exact letter shape, it is the child's attempts to make the shapes with his body that is the valuable learning experience.

Action Alphabet "D"

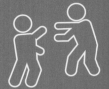

Each "Action Alphabet" activity is an independent and fun letter exploration with a short script for the teacher. An "Action Alphabet" activity can be used in conjunction with letter studies or as a simple movement and shape activity.

Explores language and literacy!

What You Need

☼ a small space

☼ "Dinosaur Romp" instrumental (disc 1, track 21)

☼ a large card showing the capital letter "D"

What You Do

Begin the letter exploration with each of the children standing in a home spot in a circle, with plenty of room between each child. During the activity, have the children return to their home spots whenever necessary. Hold up a large card showing a capital letter "D." Say to the children:

The letter "D" is made of two shapes, a straight line and a curve. Let's play a freeze game about "straight" and "curve." I'll put on some music, and you can dance while the music is playing. When I stop the music, freeze in the shape I call out. I'll call out "curve" or "straight," and then you form a curved shape or a straight one with your body.

But I'm also going to call out different levels, "high" and "low." For example, what if I stop the music and say "high curve"? Can you make a high curve with your body? Can you stretch way up on your toes and make your body into a curved shape? What about a low curve? How low can you get while making your body into a curve? Let's try "low straight" and "high straight" too.

36

There are many ways you can make these shapes. Now let's play the freeze game. Get ready for the music!

Play "Dinosaur Romp" instrumental. Conclude the activity when the song ends, with the children holding their final shape. Say:

Look around at all the different low curved shapes (for example) **the other children are making! Some children are squatting very low, others are lying on their sides on the ground, and others are lying on their backs, curled up into a ball!**

Remember that the kinesthetic exploration of letters is what is important, not the finished product. Whether or not she accomplishes the exact letter shape, it is the child's attempts to make the shapes with her body that is the valuable learning experience.

Modifications

Prompt children who have difficulty making shapes with their whole bodies to use body parts instead. You can, for example, encourage a child to try making a curved shape with his arm, hand, or fingers.

You can ask the child to identify and hold up a picture of a straight or curved line while the other children make the same shape with their bodies. He can hold up the letter card for you and point to different parts of the letter while you instruct the other children to make the shapes. For instance, he can point to a curve while you prompt the others to make their bodies into a curved shape; this will help him develop letter recognition and be an active participant in the group.

Give the child an opportunity to call out some of the prompts in the lesson. When you stop the music for the freeze game, quietly tell him the prompt to give the children ("low straight!"), and let him call it out.

Action Alphabet
"E" and "F"

• • • • • • • • • •

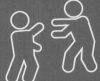

Each "Action Alphabet" activity is an independent and fun letter exploration with a short script for the teacher. An "Action Alphabet" activity can be used in conjunction with letter studies or as a simple movement and shape activity. Because these two letters are very similar, the movement studies have been grouped together, although each one can be used separately as well, by using the parts of the study pertaining to the specific letter. This alphabet activity is similar to Activity 44: Action Alphabet "M" and "N."

Explores language and literacy!

What You Need

☼ a small space (the free dance at the end of the activity can be done in place in a home spot or moving throughout a large, unobstructed space)

☼ "Follow Game" instrumental (disc 2, track 22)

☼ a large card showing the capital letters "E" and "F"

What You Do

Begin the letter exploration with each of the children standing in a home spot in a circle, with plenty of room between each child. During the activity, have the children return to their home spots whenever necessary. Hold up a large card showing a capital letter "E" and a capital letter "F." Say to the children:

The letters "E" and "F" are made up of straight lines. Can you see how many straight lines are in the letter "E"? Let's count them together:

37

one, two, three, four! Now let's count the straight lines in the letter "F." There are three! "F" is just like "E" except it doesn't have the line along the bottom of the letter.

Make your body into a straight line. As you stand straight, think of a part of your body you can use to make another straight shape. Now think of a different one. Are there any more?

When I clap my hands, I want you to pick a body part and make it straight. Repeat this several times. **Now when I clap, make two body parts straight at the same time. For example, make your body a tall straight line with your arms tight by your sides, then lift one arm out in front of you. Your body makes one line, and your arm makes another!**

Repeat the task of making two straight lines several times. Discourage the children from using just their fingers during this part of the activity, which is intended to be a whole-body kinesthetic experience.

Next we will try to make three parts straight at the same time. Try holding one arm out in front of you and the other one out to the side. Your body is one line, and each of your arms makes different straight lines. Let's try three straight lines another way. Standing tall, lift your leg to the front and hold it. Now take one arm out to the side. Do you see the three straight lines? Your body, your leg, and your arm each make a different straight line. Can you try again and make three straight lines another way? Repeat this a few times.

Let's try to make four body parts straight at the same time! First let's try a balancing shape. Demonstrate this first, and count your straight lines for the children. **Stand tall, and lift one leg behind you just off the floor. Lift one arm to the front, and one to the side. Your body and standing leg make one line, your leg to the back makes another, and your two arms make two more straight lines! Now let's try a jumping shape with four straight lines. Holding your arms in a "V" shape, jump, and lift both legs out to the side. Your arms make two straight lines, and your legs make two straight lines!** Repeat this a few times.

You're using your body to make straight lines in many directions. The letter "E" also uses four straight lines. How can we use four straight lines to make the "E" shape with our bodies? Let's sit down in our circle to do this part of the activity.

Place your feet out in front of you. Now put one arm straight out in front of you, and put the other one straight out in front but higher up. You've made an "E"! You have four straight lines in your body: your upper body is one, your legs are another, and each of your arms makes a straight line. Look around the circle at all of the other children making the "E" shapes with their bodies!

Let's lie down and make an upside down "E." Keeping your feet together, lift your legs straight up in the air and hold them there while you place your arms. Lift one arm, reaching straight over your head, and lift the other one slightly forward of the first, toward your legs. We've made lots of upside down "E"s!

Now let's stand up and make the "F" shape with our bodies. I'll demonstrate. First I stand very tall. I put one arm straight down by my side and one arm straight out in front of me. I hold this, and then I lift up my leg so it's straight out in front of me. Can you do this too? Try to keep your balance! Now carefully look around. Everyone is making their bodies into the letter "F"!

If you kneel and put one arm straight out in front of you, and put the other one straight out in front but higher up, you can make the letter "F" another way!

Let's finish this activity with a free dance about the letters "E" and "F." Play "Follow Game" instrumental. Think about making many straight lines with many different parts of your body, and also about making many "E" and "F" shapes. When the music is finished, make your body into a great big letter "E" or "F" shape!

If you have room, allow the children to move around in the larger space. If not, ask them to dance in a home spot.

Remember that the kinesthetic exploration of letters is what is important, not the finished product. Whether or not he accomplishes the exact letter shape, it is the child's attempts to make the shapes with his body that is the valuable learning experience.

Modifications

Prompt children who have difficulty making shapes with their whole bodies to use body parts instead. You can, for example, encourage a child to try making a straight line with her arm, hand, or fingers.

You can ask the child to identify and hold up a picture of a straight line while the other children make the same shape with their bodies. She can hold up the letter card for you and point to different parts of the letter while you instruct the other children to make the shapes. For instance, the child can point to a straight line while you prompt the others to make their bodies into a straight line; this will help her develop letter recognition and be an active participant in the group.

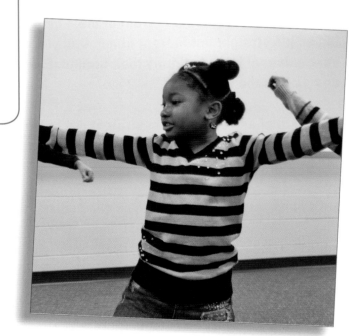

Action Alphabet "G"

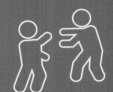

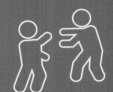

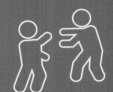
38

Each "Action Alphabet" activity is an independent and fun letter exploration with a short script for the teacher. An "Action Alphabet" activity can be used in conjunction with letter studies or as a simple movement and shape activity. This alphabet activity is similar to Activity 46: Action Alphabet "R."

> **Explores language and literacy!**

What You Need

☼ a small space (the free dance at the end of the activity can be done in place in a home spot or moving throughout a large, unobstructed space)

☼ "Goldie Rock" instrumental (disc 2, track 23)

☼ chalk, small nonslip mats, or masking tape

What You Do

On the floor, lay out a large capital "G" about four- to six-feet long. If you have a rug, you can create the letter shape using chalk or small mats. If you don't have a rug, you can create the letter shape using masking tape, chalk, or nonslip mats. Say to the children:

Today we will learn about the shape of the letter "G." As you can see, the letter "G" is made up of a curve and one straight line. Let's sit in a circle around the big letter. I'll walk the path of the "G" first. Demonstrate the path.

When I call your name, I'd like each of you to walk the path of the letter. You can use forward steps or backward steps. Begin at the top of the curve, and finish at the end of the straight line.

If the children are still engaged, ask them to take another turn using different steps, such as side steps or baby steps.

Now that you've walked the path of the letter "G," with its big curved line and small straight line, let's try making those shapes with our bodies while we're moving. When I put the music on, let's dance about the path of the letter "G," and the straight and curved lines in the letter.

Play "Goldie Rock" instrumental. If you have room, allow the children to move around in the larger space. If not, ask them to dance in a home spot. When the music comes to an end, ask the children to freeze in a "G" shape.

Remember that the kinesthetic exploration of letters is what is important, not the finished product. Whether or not she accomplishes the exact letter shape, it is the child's attempts to make the shapes with her body that is the valuable learning experience.

Modifications

Prompt children who have difficulty making shapes with their whole bodies to use body parts instead. You can, for example, encourage a child to try making a curved shape with his arm, hand, or fingers.

You can also ask him to hold up the letter card and trace the outline of the "G" shape while the other children are walking the path. This can help him develop letter recognition and be an active participant in the group.

Action Alphabet "H"

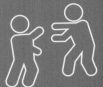

Each "Action Alphabet" activity is an independent and fun letter exploration with a short script for the teacher. An "Action Alphabet" activity can be used in conjunction with letter studies or as a simple movement and shape activity. This alphabet activity is a good lead-in to Activity 83: The Dancing Letter "H."

Explores language and literacy!

What You Need

☼ a small space

☼ a large card showing the capital letter "H"

What You Do

Begin the letter exploration with each of the children standing in a home spot in a circle, with plenty of room between each child. During the activity, have the children return to their home spots whenever necessary. Hold up a large card showing a capital letter "H." Say to the children:

Let's take a look at the letter "H." How many straight lines are in the "H"? Three! Two children at a time, we're going to learn to make this letter with our bodies. Select two children to come to the center of the circle.

I'd like the two of you to stand tall and face each other, just like the two big lines in the letter "H." Now bring your arms up in front of you and join your hands. Look everyone! Can you see the big letter "H" these two have formed?

Now let's move! Will the two of you move very slowly in a small circle and see if you can keep the big letter H shape the whole time? Now turn around the other way, stopping in the places where you began.

39

Can you both stand on your tiptoes while holding the shape? Can you first bend your knees, and then jump while you're in the letter "H" shape? Five times in a row? Can you hop? Try three times hopping on one foot, then three times on the other foot.

Give each pair of children a chance to make and move as the letter "H" in the center of the circle while the others watch. Then ask each of the pairs to make their "H" again, all at the same time. A little space between the pairs is sufficient. Say:

Can you squat and make a low "H" together? Can you stand on your tiptoes? Let's repeat that—low, high, low, high!

Modifications

Prompt children who have difficulty making shapes with their whole bodies to use body parts instead. You can, for example, encourage a child to try making the "H" shape with her arm, hand, or fingers.

You can ask the child to identify and hold up a picture of a straight line while the other children make the same shape with their bodies. She can hold up the letter card for you and point to different parts of the letter "H" while you instruct the other children to make the shapes. For instance, she can point to a straight line while you prompt the others to make their bodies into a straight line; this will help her develop letter recognition and be an active participant in the group.

Let's all make hopping "H"s at the same time. I will count to four, and each of you hop on one foot while holding your "H" shape. Change feet, and hop again. Now let's all do eight high jumps! Freeze on the landing of your last jump, in your big "H" shape!

Remember that the kinesthetic exploration of letters is what is important, not the finished product. Whether or not he accomplishes the exact letter shape, it is the child's attempts to make the shapes with his body that is the valuable learning experience.

Action Alphabet "I"

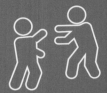

Each "Action Alphabet" activity is an independent and fun letter exploration with a short script for the teacher. An "Action Alphabet" activity can be used in conjunction with letter studies or as a simple movement and shape activity.

Explores language and literacy!

What You Need

☼ a small space

☼ "Kweezletown" instrumental (disc 2, track 27)

☼ a large card showing the capital letter "I"

What You Do

Begin the letter exploration with each of the children standing in a home spot in a circle, with plenty of room between each child. During the activity, have the children return to their home spots whenever necessary. Hold up a large card showing a capital letter "I." Say to the children:

The letter "I" is both a letter and a word. "I" is the word we use when we talk about ourselves. The letter "I" is made of a long straight line and two short straight lines, one that crosses the top of the long line and one that crosses the bottom. We can make the letter "I" out of our bodies with a little added imagination.

First, stand very straight! Now turn your feet out so your toes point away from your body; this shape is the short line at the bottom of the letter. For the top line of the "I," imagine you have a big book balancing on top of your head. Be careful! Don't let it fall off! You'll have to stand very straight and tall to keep it balanced. With your straight body, your feet pointing out, and an imaginary book on your head, you are making the letter "I"!

40

Now let's listen to some music and see if we can carefully move around the room in our "I" shapes. Play "Kweezletown" instrumental. **Hold your arms close to your sides to make a long straight line. Keep your toes pointed out, and don't let the book fall off your head as you move around. Remember that everyone else is doing the same thing, so walk carefully!**

Suggest movement variations as the children travel around the room:

- **Try to turn around with the imaginary book on your head.**

- **Now try going up on your tiptoes. Can you walk on your tiptoes?**

- **Now go back to regular walking. Can you walk in slow motion? Now can you walk faster and still balance your book?**

- **Walk back to your home spot, and bend forward to let the imaginary book drop off of your head. Catch it with your hands!**

Modifications

Prompt children who have difficulty making shapes with their whole bodies to use body parts instead. You can, for example, encourage a child to try making a straight line with his arm, hand, or fingers.

You can ask him to identify and hold up a picture of a straight line while the other children make the same shape with their bodies. He can hold up the letter card for you and point to different parts of the letter while you instruct the other children to make the shapes. For instance, he can point to a straight line while you prompt the others to make their bodies into a straight line; this will help him develop letter recognition and be an active participant in the group.

Remember that the kinesthetic exploration of letters is what is important, not the finished product. Whether or not she accomplishes the exact letter shape, it is the child's attempts to make the shapes with her body that is the valuable learning experience.

Action Alphabet "J"

Each "Action Alphabet" activity is an independent and fun letter exploration with a short script for the teacher. An "Action Alphabet" activity can be used in conjunction with letter studies or as a simple movement and shape activity.

Explores language and literacy!

What You Need

☼ a small space

☼ a large card showing the capital letter "J"

What You Do

Begin the letter exploration with each of the children standing in a home spot in a circle, with plenty of room between each child. During the activity, have the children return to their home spots whenever necessary. Hold up a large card showing a capital letter "J." Say to the children:

The letter "J" looks like an upside-down candy cane, doesn't it? Can you make a candy cane shape with your body while you're standing up? Now can you get down on the floor and make another candy cane shape? Try it on your back, then on each side, and then try it sitting. There are many ways to make a "J" shape with your body while you're on the floor.

I'm going to clap my hands five times. On the first clap, let's get up on our feet and make a standing "J." On the second clap, let's go back down to the floor and make a floor "J." We'll keep alternating until we get to the fifth clap. Freeze in that last standing "J" shape!

Remember that the kinesthetic exploration of letters is what is important, not the finished product. Whether or not he accomplishes the exact letter shape, it is the child's attempts to make the shapes with his body that is the valuable learning experience.

Modifications

Prompt children who have difficulty making shapes with their whole bodies to use body parts instead. You can, for example, encourage a child to try making a curved shape with his arm, hand, or fingers.

You can ask the child to identify and hold up a picture of a curved line while the other children make the same shape with their bodies. She can hold up the letter card for you and point to different parts of the letter while you instruct the other children to make the shapes. For instance, she can point to a curve while you prompt the others to make their bodies into a curved shape; this will help her develop letter recognition and be an active participant in the group.

Give the child an opportunity to call out some of the prompts in the lesson. For example, she can clap along with you as the children are going from their standing "J"s to their floor "J"s.

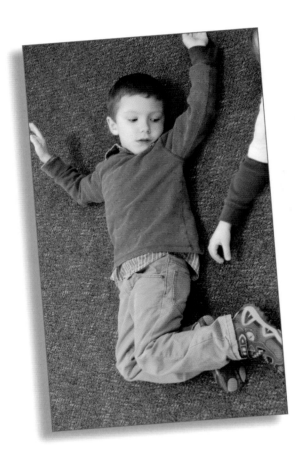

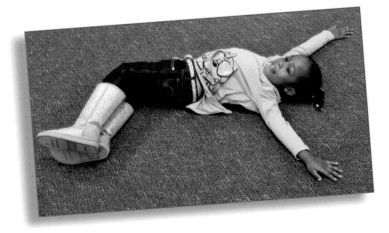

Action Alphabet "K"

Each "Action Alphabet" activity is an independent and fun letter exploration with a short script for the teacher. An "Action Alphabet" activity can be used in conjunction with letter studies or as a simple movement and shape activity.

What You Need

Explores language and literacy!

☼ a small space

☼ a large card showing the capital letter "K"

What You Do

Begin the letter exploration with each of the children standing in a home spot in a circle, with plenty of room between each child. During the activity, have the children return to their home spots whenever necessary. Hold up a large card showing a capital letter "K." Say to the children:

The letter "K" is made up of straight lines. How many straight lines do you see? Let's begin by lying down on our backs. Make your body very straight, just like the long straight line of the letter "K." Now lift your arms together and reach them up to the ceiling. You've made the second straight line of the "K." Last, lift one of your legs toward the ceiling—this makes the third straight line in the letter "K." Now bend your arms and leg! This isn't how the letter "K" is, right? Now straighten them again to make the "K" correctly. Let's bend and straighten our arms and leg several times. Do you feel the difference between the bent lines and the straight lines?

Now let's stand up and try the "K" shape standing. Stand up very straight. This is the first straight line. Next extend your arms out in front of you like I'm doing (hold your arms a little higher than parallel to the floor)—**this**

42

is the second straight line. For the last straight line, slide one leg out in front of you and lift it a little so just your toes are touching the floor while you stand and balance on the other leg. Can you hold this shape? For how long? Let's make all three straight lines bend, just like we did on the floor: bend, straight, bend, straight. Let's see if we can make our "K" shape turn. Take little tiny hops on your standing leg to turn, and try to hold that nice "K" shape. Try it turning in the other direction.

Modifications

Prompt children who have difficulty making shapes with their whole bodies to use body parts instead. You can, for example, encourage a child to try making a straight line with his arm, hand, or fingers.

You can ask him to identify and hold up a picture of a straight line while the other children make the same shape with their bodies. He can hold up the letter card for you and point to different parts of the letter while you instruct the other children to make the shapes. For instance, the child can point to the straight lines while you prompt the others to make their bodies into the straight lines of the letter "K"; this will help him develop letter recognition and be an active participant in the group.

Repeat this part of the exercise using the other leg as the standing leg: make the shape, bend and straighten all three lines, and turn around in a little circle. Finish by making one last "K" shape on the floor.

Remember that the kinesthetic exploration of letters is what is important, not the finished product. Whether or not she accomplishes the exact letter shape, it is the child's attempts to make the shapes with her body that is the valuable learning experience.

Action Alphabet "L"

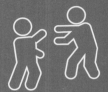

Each "Action Alphabet" activity is an independent and fun letter exploration with a short script for the teacher. An "Action Alphabet" activity can be used in conjunction with letter studies or as a simple movement and shape activity.

What You Need

Explores language and literacy!

☼ a small space

☼ "Care of the Earth" instrumental (disc 1, track 16)

☼ a large card showing the capital letter "L"

What You Do

Begin the letter exploration with each of the children standing in a home spot in a circle, with plenty of room between each child. During the activity, have the children return to their home spots whenever necessary. Say to the children:

Let's all sit down in our circle. Put your feet out in front of you. Do you see the shape your body is making? There is a straight line in your body, and then a straight line from your hips to your toes. Look at this picture of the letter "L." Hold up a large card showing a capital letter "L." **We're all making the same shape with our bodies! Can you make that shape using both of your arms, with one straight up and one straight forward? Now change and make it with your other arm up. Switch back and forth from one "L" to another while you sit in the "L" shape!**

Now lie down on your back, and bring your legs straight up in the air. We're making an upside-down "L"! Can you roll onto your side and make an "L" shape on your side? Do the same thing on the other side!

43

Sit up, and we'll open our circle into a line. I'll be the leader. Sit in the "L" shape with your feet out in front of you, and make sure your feet aren't touching the person in front of you. We're a long line of "L" shapes! The words "long" and "line" begin with "L."

Now that we're in a long line, let's imagine we're in a rowboat. Everyone begin rowing! I'll play the music (play "Care of the Earth" instrumental), and we'll row across a lake! Can you hear the sound the word "lake" starts with? Keep rowing until we get all the way across the lake!

Remember that the kinesthetic exploration of letters is what is important, not the finished product. Whether or not he accomplishes the exact letter shape, it is the child's attempts to make the shapes with his body that is the valuable learning experience.

Modifications

Prompt children who have difficulty making shapes with their whole bodies to use body parts instead. You can, for example, encourage a child to try making a straight line with his arm, hand, or fingers.

You can ask the child to identify and hold up a picture of a straight line while the other children make the same shape with their bodies. She can hold up the letter card for you and point to different parts of the letter while you instruct the other children to make the shapes. For instance, she can point to a straight line while you prompt the others to make their bodies into a straight line; this will help her develop letter recognition and be an active participant in the group.

She can also participate in the last part of the activity by rowing along to the music, whether or not she is sitting in the line with the other children.

Action Alphabet "M" and "N"

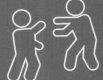

Each "Action Alphabet" activity is an independent and fun letter exploration with a short script for the teacher. An "Action Alphabet" activity can be used in conjunction with letter studies or as a simple movement and shape activity. Because these two letters are very similar, the movement studies have been grouped together, although each one can be used separately as well, by using the parts of the study pertaining to each specific letter. This alphabet activity is similar to Activity 37: Action Alphabet "E" and "F."

Explores language and literacy!

What You Need

☼ a small space (the free dance at the end of the activity can be done in place in a home spot or by moving throughout a large, unobstructed space)

☼ "Shine & Brighten" instrumental (disc 2, track 37)

☼ a large card showing the capital letters "M" and "N"

What You Do

Begin the letter exploration with each of the children standing in a home spot in a circle, with plenty of room between each child. During the activity, have the children return to their home spots whenever necessary. Hold up a large card showing a capital letter "M" and a capital letter "N." Say to the children:

The letters "M" and "N" are made up of straight lines. Can you see how many straight lines are in the letter "M"? Let's count them

44

together: one, two, three, four! Now let's count the straight lines in the letter "N." There are three!

Make your body into a straight line. As you stand straight, think of a part of your body you can use to make another straight shape. Now think of different one. Are there any more?

When I clap my hands, I want you to pick a body part and make it straight. Repeat this several times. **Now when I clap, make two body parts straight at the same time. For example, make your body a tall straight line with your arms tight by your sides, then lift one arm out in front of you. Your body makes one line, and your arm makes another!**

Repeat the task of making two straight lines several times. Discourage the children from using just their fingers during this part of the activity, which is intended to be a whole-body kinesthetic experience.

Next we will try to make three parts straight at the same time. Try holding one arm out in front of you and the other one out to the side. Your body is one line, and each of your arms makes a different straight line. Let's try three straight lines another way. Standing tall, with your arms at your sides, lift your leg to the front and hold it. Now take one arm out to the side. Do you see the three straight lines? Your body, your leg, and your arm each make a different straight line. Can you try again making three straight lines another way? Repeat this a few times.

Let's try to make four body parts straight at the same time! First let's try a balancing shape. Demonstrate this first, and count your straight lines for the children. **Stand tall, and take one leg behind you in the air. Lift one arm to the front and one to the side. Your body and standing leg make one line, your leg to the back makes another, and your two arms make two more straight lines!**

Now let's try a jumping shape with four straight lines. Holding your arms in a "V" shape, jump and lift both legs out to the side. Your arms make two straight lines, and your legs make two straight lines. You're using your body to make straight lines in many directions! Repeat this a few times.

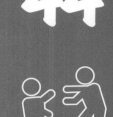

The letter "M" also uses four straight lines. How can we use four straight lines to make the "M" shape with our bodies? Let's try the "M" shape while standing, kneeling, and lying down.

The children may or may not accomplish the "M" shape exactly, but it's the exploration and attempt to make the shape that's important.

Let's try to make the "N" shape with our bodies too—standing, sitting, kneeling, and lying down. Remember, the "N" shape is made of three straight lines! Let's count the straight lines on this letter one more time. Can you try it standing? Now let's try it sitting, kneeling, and then lying down.

Let's finish this activity with a free dance about the letters "M" and "N." Think about making straight lines with many different parts of your body. Also think about making many different "M" and "N" shapes.

Play "Shine & Brighten" instrumental. If you have room, allow the children to move around in the larger space. If not, ask them to dance in a home spot. Let them finish the dance by making their bodies into a great big letter "M" or "N."

Remember that the kinesthetic exploration of letters is what is important, not the finished product. Whether or not she accomplishes the exact letter shape, it is the child's attempts to make the shapes with her body that is the valuable learning experience.

Modifications

Prompt children who have difficulty making shapes with their whole bodies to use body parts instead. You can, for example, encourage a child to try making a straight line with his arm, hand, or fingers.

You can ask the child to identify and hold up a picture of a straight line while the other children make the same shape with their bodies. He can hold up the letter card for you and point to different parts of the letter while you instruct the other children to make the shapes. For instance, he can point to a straight line while you prompt the others to make their bodies into a straight line; this will help him develop letter recognition and be an active participant in the group.

45

Action Alphabet "O," "P," and "Q"

● ● ● ● ● ● ● ● ● ● ● ● ●

Each "Action Alphabet" activity is an independent and fun letter exploration with a short script for the teacher. An "Action Alphabet" activity can be used in conjunction with letter studies or as a simple movement and shape activity. Because these three letters have some similar qualities, the movement studies have been grouped together, although each one can be used separately as well by using the parts of the study pertaining to each specific letter.

Explores language and literacy!

What You Need

☼ a small space (the free dance at the end of the activity can be done in place in a home spot or by moving throughout a large, unobstructed space)

☼ "Pelican" instrumental (disc 2, track 34)

☼ a large card showing the capital letters "O," "P," and "Q"

What You Do

Begin the letter exploration with each of the children standing in a home spot in a circle, with plenty of room between each child. During the activity, have the children return to their home spots whenever necessary. Hold up a large card showing a capital letter "O," "P," and "Q." Say to the children:

All three of these letters have circles in them. Can you see that the letter "O" is just one great big circle? Everyone lie down and make

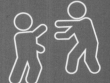

your whole body into a circle. Try it while you are lying on your back, and then while you are lying on your side, then on your other side. Now let's try it sitting. Now try it another way while you are sitting! Can you try to make yourself into a great big "O" shape while you are kneeling?

Now let's try it standing up. How many ways can you make yourself into a circular "O" shape while you are standing?

Hold up the large card again showing a capital "O," "P," and "Q" and say to the children:

Let's sit down and look again at the letter "P." What makes it different from the "O"? It has a straight line, and the "O" shape in the "P" is touching the straight line. Can you try to make a "P" with your body while lying down? Now let's try it sitting, then kneeling, and then standing up.

Hold up the large card one more time showing a capital "O," "P," and "Q" and say:

Let's look at the letter "Q" now. Can you see something that makes the letter "Q" different from the letter "O"? It has a very small straight line on it, doesn't it? Let's see if we can figure out a way to make the letter "Q" with our bodies, first lying down, then sitting, kneeling, and standing.

Let's finish the activity with a free dance about the letters "O," "P," and "Q." Play "Pelican" instrumental. While you're dancing, try to make straight lines and circles with many different parts of your body. When I stop the music, I'll call out "O," "P," or "Q," and when I do, freeze in that shape. I'll start and stop the music several times. When it's time to finish the dance, I'll say, "Freeze in a 'P' shape!" Then you can make your body into a great big letter "P"!

45

Remember that the kinesthetic exploration of letters is what is important, not the finished product. Whether or not he accomplishes the exact letter shape, it is the child's attempts to make the shapes with his body that is the valuable learning experience.

Modifications

Prompt children who have difficulty making shapes with their whole bodies to use body parts instead. You can, for example, encourage a child to try making a curved shape with her arm, hand, or fingers.

You can ask the child to identify and hold up a picture of a straight or curved line while the other children make the same shape with their bodies. She can hold up the letter card for you and point to different parts of the letter while you instruct the other children to make the shapes. For instance, she can point to a curve while you prompt the others to make their bodies into a curved shape; this will help her develop letter recognition and be an active participant in the group.

Give the child an opportunity to call out some of the prompts in the lesson. She can choose the letters that are called out during the freezes in the free dance—"O!" "P!" or "Q!"

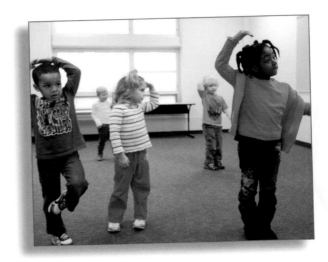

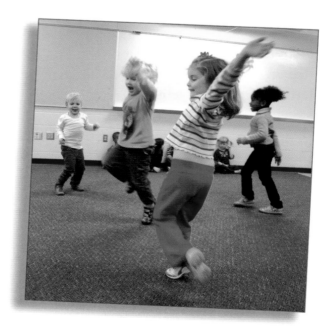

Action Alphabet "R"

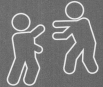

Each "Action Alphabet" activity is an independent and fun letter exploration with a short script for the teacher. An "Action Alphabet" activity can be used in conjunction with letter studies or as a simple movement and shape activity. This alphabet activity is similar to Activity 38: Action Alphabet "G."

Explores language and literacy!

What You Need

☼ a small space (the free dance at the end of the activity can be done in place in a home spot or moving throughout a large, unobstructed space)

☼ "Dance S'More" instrumental (disc 1, track 20)

☼ chalk, small nonslip mats, or masking tape

What You Do

On the floor, lay out a large capital "R" about four- to six-feet long. If you have a rug, you can create the letter shape using chalk or small mats. If you don't have a rug, you can create the letter shape using masking tape, chalk, or nonslip mats. Say to the children:

Today we will learn about the shape of the letter "R." As you can see, the letter "R" is made of a curve and two straight lines. Let's sit in a circle around the big letter. I'll walk the path of the "R" first. Demonstrate the path.

When I call your name, I'd like each of you to walk the path of the letter. You can use forward steps or backward steps. Begin at the top of the tall straight line, walk to the bottom of the line, then turn around

46

and walk back to the top. From there, follow the whole curve, and finish by walking the path of the smaller straight line.

If the children are still engaged, ask them to take another turn using different steps, such as side steps or baby steps.

Now that you've walked the path of the letter "R," with its big straight line, curved line, and small straight line, let's try making those shapes with our bodies while we're moving. When I put the music on, let's dance about the path of the letter "R," and the straight and curved lines in the letter.

Modifications

Prompt children who have difficulty making shapes with their whole bodies to use body parts instead. You can, for example, encourage a child to try making a curved shape with his arm, hand, or fingers.

You can also ask him to hold up the letter card and trace the outline of the "R" shape while the other children are walking the path. This will help him develop letter recognition and be an active participant in the group.

Play "Dance S'More." If you have room, allow the children to move around in the larger space. If not, ask them to dance in a home spot. When the music comes to an end, ask the children to freeze in an "R" shape.

Remember that the kinesthetic exploration of letters is what is important, not the finished product. Whether or not she accomplishes the exact letter shape, it is the child's attempts to make the shapes with her body that is the valuable learning experience.

Action Alphabet "S"

Each "Action Alphabet" activity is an independent and fun letter exploration with a short script for the teacher. An "Action Alphabet" activity can be used in conjunction with letter studies or as a simple movement and shape activity.

What You Need

Explores language and literacy!

☼ a small space

☼ a large card showing the capital letter "S"

What You Do

Begin the letter exploration with each of the children standing in a home spot in a circle, with plenty of room between each child. During the activity, have the children return to their home spots whenever necessary. Hold up a large card showing a capital letter "S." Say to the children:

The letter "S" looks like a squiggly, slithery, squirmy snake! And all those words start with "S"! Can you say that with me, and listen for the "S" sound? "Squiggly, slithery, squirmy snake!" That also sounds a bit like the sound a snake makes, doesn't it? Let's all say, "The squiggly, slithery, squirmy snake goes hisssssss!"

Look at the shape of the letter "S" very carefully. Let's all lie down on the floor and try to make our bodies into that shape. Can you make another "S" shape on the floor? Try it on one side, the other side, lying facedown, and lying on your back.

Next let's come up to a kneeling position and try it—make an "S" shape while kneeling. How about sitting? Can you make yourself into a squiggly "S" shape while sitting? Now let's try it standing.

47

Last, let's try something really fun. **Can you make an "S" shape with your body in the air while you are jumping? Make another silly "S" shape while jumping! Can you do it four times in a row? We will finish our game by lying on the floor in an "S" shape, and let's all say "hisssssss!"**

Modifications

Prompt children who have difficulty making shapes with their whole bodies to use body parts instead. You can, for example, encourage a child to try making a curved shape with her arm, hand, or fingers.

You can ask her to identify and hold up a picture of a curved line while the other children make the same shape with their bodies. She can hold up the letter card for you and point to different parts of the letter while you instruct the other children to make the shapes. For instance, she can point to a curve while you prompt the others to make their bodies into a curved shape; this will help her develop letter recognition and be an active participant in the group.

Give the child an opportunity to call out some of the prompts in the lesson. The child can help you call out the words "squiggly, slithery, squirmy snake," or some of the other prompts: "Try making an 'S' shape in the air!"

Remember that the kinesthetic exploration of letters is what is important, not the finished product. Whether or not he accomplishes the exact letter shape, it is the child's attempts to make the shapes with his body that is the valuable learning experience.

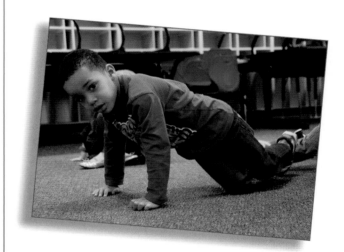

Action Alphabet "T"

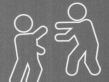

Each "Action Alphabet" activity is an independent and fun letter exploration with a short script for the teacher. An "Action Alphabet" activity can be used in conjunction with letter studies or as a simple movement and shape activity. "Action Alphabet 'T'" helps children distinguish between vertical and horizontal lines by making the different lines with their bodies.

What You Need

☼ a small space

☼ a large card showing the capital letter "T"

Explores language and literacy!

What You Do

Begin the letter exploration with each of the children standing in a home spot in a circle, with plenty of room between each child. During the activity, have the children return to their home spots whenever necessary. Hold up a large card showing a capital letter "T." Say to the children:

How many lines are in the letter "T"? One of the lines goes up and down, and one of the lines goes side to side. Let's think about those two lines and how we can make them with our bodies. Can you think of a straight line that goes up and down? Yes! We are all standing straight and tall, making a big up-and-down line. Can you make some more up-and-down lines?

Think about the straight lines of your legs. Can you stand on one leg, straight and tall? How about the other one? Now can you use your arms to make straight lines up and down? Reach one arm high above your head, then the other one, and then both together. Now try making

48

up-and-down lines with your arms, legs, and body while you're sitting, and then while you're kneeling.

Think about the side-to-side line across the top of the "T." What lines can we make with our bodies that go side to side? Can you try making some side-to-side lines in your body while standing, then sitting, and then kneeling?

Now stand up and make your whole body into a "T." Hold your "T" shape and turn around. Can you turn around the other way? Can you turn around faster? Can you hop and jump and still hold your "T" shape? Hold your "T" shape and see if you can melt to the floor, and end up in that shape on the floor as a finishing position.

Remember that the kinesthetic exploration of letters is what is important, not the finished product. Whether or not she accomplishes the exact letter shape, it is the child's attempts to make the shapes with her body that is the valuable learning experience.

Modifications

Prompt children who have difficulty making shapes with their whole bodies to use body parts instead. You can, for example, encourage a child to try making a straight line with his arm, hand, or fingers.

You can ask the child to identify and hold up a picture of a straight line while the other children make the same shape with their bodies. He can hold up the letter card for you and point to different parts of the letter while you instruct the other children to make the shapes. For instance, he can point to a straight line while you prompt the others to make their bodies into a straight line; this will help him develop letter recognition and be an active participant in the group.

Action Alphabet "U," "V," and "W"

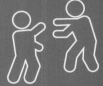

Each "Action Alphabet" activity is an independent and fun letter exploration with a short script for the teacher. An "Action Alphabet" activity can be used in conjunction with letter studies or as a simple movement and shape activity. Because these three letters have some similar qualities, the movement studies have been grouped together, although each one can be used separately as well, by using the parts of the study pertaining to each specific letter.

What You Need

Explores language and literacy!

☼ a small space

☼ large cards showing the capital letters "U," "V," and "W" (one letter per card)

What You Do

Begin the letter exploration with each of the children standing in a home spot in a circle, with plenty of room between each child. During the activity, have the children return to their home spots whenever necessary. Hold up the large cards showing the capital letters "U" and "V." Say to the children:

Let's take a look at the letters "U" and "V." Their shapes are similar, with one big difference. Can you see the difference? "V" is made of two straight lines, and "U" is made of one big curve. Let's see if we can feel these differences in our bodies!

Can you make your whole body into a "U"? You can try it standing, sitting, lying down on your back, or lying on your side. Now see if you

49

can change your "U" shape into a "V" shape by changing the big curve of the "U" into the angle of the "V." Now try to make a different "U" shape. Can you turn that one into a "V"? Let's try one more "U" shape and then change it into a "V."

Now hold up the large cards showing the capital letters "V" and "W" and say to the children:

Modifications

Prompt children who have difficulty making shapes with their whole bodies to use body parts instead. You can, for example, encourage a child to try making a curved shape with her arm, hand, or fingers.

You can ask the child to identify and hold up a picture of a straight or curved line while the other children make the same shape with their bodies. She can hold up the letter card for you and point to different parts of the letter while you instruct the other children to make the shapes. For instance, she can point to a curve while you prompt the others to make their bodies into a curved shape; this will help her develop letter recognition and be an active participant in the group.

Give the child an opportunity to call out some of the prompts in the lesson. The child who cannot participate in making the shapes with her body can help you call out the letters ("U," "V," and "W") during the last part of the lesson.

Now let's take a look at the difference between "V" and "W." What do you see? The "W" shape is actually two Vs next to each other! The "V" is made up of two straight lines, and the "W" is made up of four! Let's count them together as I point to each one.

Let's try this with our bodies. Can you try to make a "W" shape with your body while lying down? The "W" shape is fairly complex, but the children will use their imaginations as they try to recreate it. **How about when sitting? Let's try it standing.**

I will call out "U," "V," or "W" now, and you try to make each one as I do. You can make the shape lying down, sitting, kneeling, standing, or jumping!

Remember that the kinesthetic exploration of letters is what is important, not the finished product. Whether or not he accomplishes the exact letter shape, it is the child's attempts to make the shapes with his body that is the valuable learning experience.

Action Alphabet
"X," "Y," and "Z"

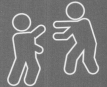

Each "Action Alphabet" activity is an independent and fun letter exploration with a short script for the teacher. An "Action Alphabet" activity can be used in conjunction with letter studies or as a simple movement and shape activity. Because these three letters have some similar qualities, the movement studies have been grouped together, although each one can be used separately as well by using the parts of the study pertaining to each specific letter.

Explores language and literacy!

What You Need

☼ a small space (the free dance at the end of the activity can be done in place in a home spot or moving throughout a large, unobstructed space)

☼ "Higgeldy Dance" instrumental (disc 2, track 25)

☼ large cards showing the capital letters "X," "Y," and "Z" (one letter per card)

What You Do

Begin the letter exploration with each of the children standing in a home spot in a circle, with plenty of room between each child. During the activity, have the children return to their home spots whenever necessary. Hold up large cards showing the capital letters "X," "Y," and "Z." Say to the children:

Let's take a look at the letters "X," "Y," and "Z." These are the last three letters of the alphabet, and they're all made up of straight lines! When I

hold up one of these three letters, try to make its shape with your body. You can make the letter shape lying down, sitting, kneeling, standing, or up in the air! Show the different cards several times in a random order.

Now let's dance about these three letters. Play "Higgeldy Dance" instrumental. **You can leave your home spot and dance freely. When I hold up one of the letters, freeze in that letter shape. Watch me carefully so you know when to freeze!**

Repeat the freeze several times using the letters in random order. Finish the dance by asking the children to freeze in one of the letter shapes.

Remember that the kinesthetic exploration of letters is what is important, not the finished product. Whether or not she accomplishes the exact letter shape, it is the child's attempts to make the shapes with her body that is the valuable learning experience.

Modifications

Prompt children who have difficulty making shapes with their whole bodies to use body parts instead. You can, for example, encourage a child to try making a straight line with his arm, hand, or fingers.

You can ask him to identify and hold up a picture of a straight line while the other children make the same shape with their bodies. He can hold up the letter card for you and point to different parts of the letter while you instruct the other children to make the shapes. For instance, he can point to a straight line while you prompt the others to make their bodies into a straight line; this will help him develop letter recognition and be an active participant in the group.

Give the child an opportunity to call out some of the prompts in the lesson. The child who cannot participate in making the shapes with his body could call out the letters ("X," "Y," and "Z") or hold up the cards during the free dance.

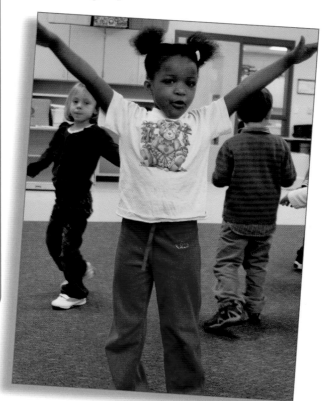

Word Rhythms

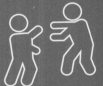

"Word Rhythms" is a movement activity that helps children become familiar with the sounds of syllables. With simple adaptations, it can also be used to address a theme or to help children become familiar with different categories or patterns.

Explores language and literacy!

What You Need

☼ a small space (the free dance at the end of the activity can be done in place in a home spot or moving throughout a large, unobstructed space)

What You Do

Begin the activity with the children sitting in a home spot in a circle. Say to the children:

Today we are going to talk about the names of some of the fruits we like to eat. I will begin with "apple." The word "apple" has two sounds, a loud clap and a quieter clap. Let's clap the rhythm of "apple" while we say the word: "ap-ple." Let's try it now with just the claps.

Now let's try another fruit: "banana." "Banana" has three sounds. Let's clap it while saying the word: "Ba-na-na" (clap one time quietly, one time loudly, and once more quietly), **and then do the claps without the word.**

Let's put them together now—let's clap the rhythm of "apple," and then let's clap the rhythm of "banana."

"Watermelon" has four sounds. Let's try that one next: wa-ter-mel-on. Say the word and clap the rhythm. Then try all three words together,

clapping and saying: "ap-ple, ba-na-na, wa-ter-mel-on." Try it again, clapping the rhythm without saying the words.

Let's end our rhythm sentence with the word "grape," which is a strong ending: "grape!" Put the word and the clap together. Next let's try our whole rhythm sentence with the words and clapping: "ap-ple, ba-na-na, wa-ter-mel-on, grape!" Let's try it with only the clapping now. Wow! We've made a sentence with word rhythms!

Have the children practice until they can clap the whole series of words—apple, banana, watermelon, grape!—without needing to say the words aloud to maintain the rhythm. Then suggest variations to the tempo:

- **Can we clap the rhythm very slowly?**

- **Can we clap it faster together?**

Next the children should try to express the rhythm using other body parts—nodding their heads, tapping their toes, lifting and lowering their shoulders. Say to the children:

Now we'll stand up. Let's think of ways we can make the rhythms with our whole bodies. Can we make the rhythm with our feet, instead of clapping? While we're doing that, let's move around, and for the last word, "grape!" let's all do a big jump.

If you have room, allow the children to move around in the larger space. If not, ask them to move in a home spot.

Modifications

Children can also participate in this exercise by verbalizing and clapping the rhythms, as well as contributing words to use for the rhythm sentences.

Use this syllable and rhythm exercise again as a lesson about a theme and to explore categories and patterns. Introduce different topics, such as colors or transportation, and think of basic words from your theme. For example, for a lesson on transportation, you might use the words "airplane, helicopter, submarine, train!" You can make another one using "bicycle, bus, fire truck, car!" Invite suggestions from the children as you explore the theme, and develop them into a movement routine using the steps described above.

Can You Be a Happy Cat?

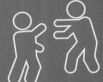

"Can You Be a Happy Cat?" is a lively activity using a poem as the prompt. The many color references and the different characteristics of cats can be used to build comprehension and vocabulary. "Can You Be a Happy Cat?" can be used as a quick movement break between other daily activities as well as between the different parts of the daily routine.

What You Need

☼ a small space

Explores language and literacy!

What You Do

Begin this activity with the children standing in a circle or in a home spot throughout the room. Recite the poem to the children. Talk about any words that are unfamiliar to the children.

Can You Be a Happy Cat?

Can you be a happy cat?
Bounce a red ball, pat, pat, pat!

Can you be a bashful cat?
Hide behind a yellow straw hat!

Can you be a silly cat?
Jump in a mud puddle, splish-kersplat!

Can you be a curious cat?
Look around for a furry gray rat!

Can you be a cartoon cat?
Stretch up tall, then make yourself flat!

52

Can you be a playful cat?
Crouch and leap and chase a gnat!

Can you be a quiet cat?
Tiptoe softly on a fuzzy blue mat!

Can you be a sleepy cat?
Yawn, stretch, purr, and that is that!

To help set the mood, ask the children to go onto their hands and knees and imagine they are cats. Prompt them with questions such as, "What color kitty are you?" and "What size kitty are you?"

Now invite the children to respond with movement to each verse in the poem as you read it again. Encourage them to come up with their own individual movement responses while remaining in their home spots. Pause after each verse to allow them to create and expand their ideas. Here are a few ideas to help the children to get started.

Can you be a happy cat?
Bounce a red ball, pat, pat, pat!

- move around home spot on hands and knees and imagine playing with a ball

Can you be a bashful cat?
Hide behind a yellow straw hat!

- curl into a ball, or bend arms and knees until body is close to floor, and hide face with arms

Can you be a silly cat?
Jump in a mud puddle, splish-kersplat!

- stand up and do one big jump

Can you be a curious cat?
Look around for a furry gray rat!

- go back down to hands and knees, move around home spot as if chasing something

Can you be a cartoon cat?
Stretch up tall, then make yourself flat!

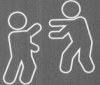

- stand up and go onto tiptoes while stretching arms high in the air, then lie down on floor and stretch with arms overhead

Can you be a playful cat?
Crouch and leap and chase a gnat!

- crouch, leap, return to crouch position, repeat three times

Can you be a quiet cat?
Tiptoe softly on a fuzzy blue mat!

- stand up, tiptoe around home spot

Can you be a sleepy cat?
Yawn, stretch, purr and that is that!

- go back down to hands and knees, stretch by arching and curving the back, sit, stretch the arms and legs, yawn and then curl up in a ball

Demonstrate the movements as you say each verse, or say the verse and then show the movement ideas. Say the verses slowly and allow children to explore each idea before moving to the next verse. Repeat the activity and allow the children to expand and explore the movement ideas.

Modifications

Invite the child to help you call out the words of the poem while the others are moving. Quietly prompt her with the words before you say each line, and then have her repeat them aloud to the group with you. If you have pictures of cats doing the various movements described above, the child can hold up a picture during the corresponding verse.

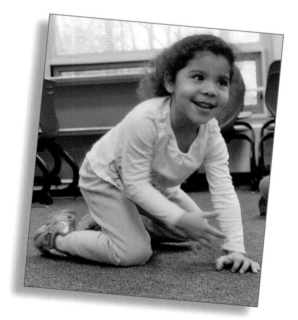

The Language of Gestures

53

This is a movement study that uses common gestures in place of words. Children will try to interpret your gesture sentence, and build their own sentences using different gestures. When they engage in this playful activity, children begin to learn about sentence structure while using large and small body movements.

> **Explores language and literacy!**

What You Need

☼ a small space (the free dance at the end of the activity can be done in place in a home spot or moving throughout the shared space)

☼ "Jambo: Hello" (disc 1, track 7)

What You Do

Sit in a circle for the beginning of this activity. Say to the children:

When we want to say something, we usually use words. But did you know that movement can be a language too? We often use movements instead of words, such as nodding instead of saying "yes" or waving instead of saying "hello." These movements are called gestures. Let's think of as many gestures as we can.

Give the children hints as they brainstorm while you demonstrate some or all of the following common gestures:

- nod your head ("Yes.")

- shake your head ("No.")

- wave your hand ("Hello." "Good-bye.")

- point your finger ("Look!")

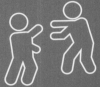

- fan your hand and fingers toward your body ("Come here.")

- shrug your shoulders ("I don't know.")

- cross your arms ("No way!")

- stomp your feet ("I'm mad!")

- hug yourself ("I'm filled with joy!")

- thumbs up ("Good job!")

- thumbs down ("Things aren't going well.")

- wink ("Hi!")

- make a V sign with your fingers ("Peace.")

- high five ("Great to see you!")

- cross your fingers ("Good luck!")

- tap your foot ("Hurry up!")

- smile ("I'm happy.")

- frown ("I'm sad")

- extend your hand from your forehead over eyes ("Where are you?")

We had a lot of ideas! These movements are called gestures. Each of these gestures is like a word. Let's try them together.

Now I'm going to put some gestures together to make a sentence—a movement sentence instead of a word sentence. You try to guess what I'm saying. Here I go!

Look sad, wave good-bye, look happy, and pretend to give someone a hug. Once the children have guessed that you are sad to say good-bye to someone, and then happy the person is coming back, hugging the person to let her know, ask the children to stand up and do the gesture phrase with you.

Here's another one—see if you can guess what I'm saying.

53

Extend your hand out from your forehead over your eyes, tap your foot, and pretend to give someone a high five, which means, "Where are you? Hurry up! Great to see you!" Once the children have guessed, ask them to do the gesture phrase with you. This one can be done with a partner; the high-five gesture becomes a clap with the other person.

Let's try one more.

Cross your arms, shake your head, and stomp your feet: "No way! I won't do it! I'm angry!" Again, once the children have guessed, ask them to perform the phrase with you.

Now let's make a gesture dance about angry and happy. First we'll do the gesture dance we just practiced: Cross your arms. Shake your head. Stomp your feet. You can even make an angry face and move your arms to show how mad you are. You all look very angry!

A very different feeling from angry is happy. I'll play a song. The song is about how children all over the world use a smile to show they're happy. Let's dance to this music and think about how our bodies move when we're happy!

Play "Jambo: Hello." If you have room, allow the children to leave the circle and move around in the larger space. If not, ask them to dance in a home spot.

Modifications

Many of the gestures, such as thumbs up and down, waving, and nodding and shaking the head, are small movements that can be done by a child who has limited mobility. Ask that child to choose the gestures he can do, and invite the other children to guess his gesture sentence.

Invite the child to sing along with the words in the song.

"Run" Rhymes with "Fun"!

"'Run' Rhymes with 'Fun'" combines an energetic, large-motor skills activity with awareness of rhyming words. The children will guess and then perform the movement that rhymes with the suggested word and also have an opportunity to develop their own pairs of rhyming words and movements.

What You Need

Explores language and literacy!

☼ a large space, indoors or outside

What You Do

With the children sitting or standing, talk briefly about what an action word is and what a rhyming word is. Say to them:

Action words describe a movement you can do, such as "climb" or "throw." Can you think of some other action words? Rhyming words are words that have similar sounds, such as these pairs of words: "climb" and "rhyme," and "throw" and "toe." Let's think of some other pairs of rhyming words.

With the children, review the following list of action words and the words that rhyme with them.

Action Word	Rhyming Word
Walk	Chalk
March	Arch
Run	Fun
Gallop	Scallop
Slide	Wide

Shake	Bake
Jump	Bump
Hop	Pop
Freeze	Please
Prance	Pants

For children ages five and up, here are two more pairs of action words and rhyming words:

Action Word	**Rhyming Word**
Skip	Dip
Leap	Deep

Now line the children up side by side, with plenty of room between each child, along the one end of the room. Say to them:

Modifications

Here are two suggestions for providing children who have limited mobility with opportunities to participate. (1) Prepare a list of smaller-motor skills activities and accompanying rhyming words (for example: write/light; pat/cat; lift/gift; blink/think; nod/pod; turn/learn; smile/style), and use it as a preliminary activity to the large-motor skills activity described above, with all of the children participating. (2) Allow the children with limited mobility to call out the words for which the other children are guessing the rhyming action words.

We're going to try some big movements across the floor, but before we do, we'll play a guessing game. I'm going to say a word, and you guess the action word that rhymes with it. Once you've guessed the right action word, you can all do that movement across to the other side of the room. Remember to slow down before you get there, so you're ready to stop when you reach the other side!

Go through the list several times, in random order.

Note that many of the action words (like "walk," "shake," "hop") have a number of words that rhyme with them. You can expand this activity by asking the children for more rhymes for certain action words or by thinking up new action words and words that rhyme with them.

Action Words in English and Spanish

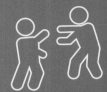

This activity is built around a poem that not only contains lots of movement prompts but also teaches some basic Spanish verbs. The playful movement facilitates and reinforces the learning of new words.

What You Need

Explores language and literacy!

☼ a large space, indoors or outside

☼ "Sunscreen" instrumental (disc 2, track 40)

☼ a world map

What You Do

Begin with the children seated in a circle. Talk to them briefly about how people in different cultures speak different languages, and point to the places on the world map where Spanish is spoken. Say to the children:

The poem I am going to read uses words from another language, Spanish. The poem tells you what the Spanish word means. Listen carefully!

There is a pronunciation guide after each of the Spanish verbs. The "r" is pronounced like a very soft "d." The double "r" in "correr" is a roll of the tongue. In all of the following verbs, the emphasis is on the second syllable.

Action Words

**I like to jump both high and far.
In Spanish it's "saltar."** (saul-*tar*)

I like to run from here to there.

In Spanish it's "correr." (core-*rare*)

I like to shine like a shooting star.
In Spanish it's "brillar." (bree-*yar*)

I like to say words loud and clear.
In Spanish it's "decir." (day-*seer*)

I like to play my new guitar.
In Spanish it's "tocar." (toe-*car*)

I like to eat a juicy pear.
In Spanish it's "comer." (ko-*mare*)

I like to laugh when friends are here.
In Spanish it's "reír." (ray-*ear*)

I like to dance like beans in a jar.
In Spanish it's "bailar." (by-*lar*)

Do you think you can guess what the words mean? What does "saltar" mean? How about "correr"?

Continue through all the Spanish words, making sure the children have a good idea of the meaning of each. Read the poem a couple of times all the way through. Ask the children to spread out in the large space and begin in a home spot. Say to them:

Now we're going to dance—"bailar"—about all the new Spanish words and the movements they describe. I will play the music. While it plays, listen carefully to my voice. I will call out one of the new Spanish words, and you will do what the word tells you. For this part of the activity, let's move around in our home spot.

Play "Sunscreen" instrumental. Use the following prompts for some of the Spanish verbs:

For "brillar" you could say: **How does it feel to be bright and shiny, like a star moving slowly or quickly across the night sky?**

For "decir" you could say: **When I say the word "decir," everyone repeat that word out loud!**

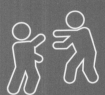

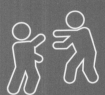

55

For "tocar" you could say: **Play air guitar!**

For "comer" you could say: **Pretend you are eating a big, juicy pear, or something else you like to eat!**

For "reír" you could say: **How do you move your body when you are laughing very hard?**

Now say to the children:

I will start the music again, and this time you can move freely throughout the space while doing what the Spanish words tell you as I call them out.
Play "Sunscreen" instrumental again.

To finish the activity, ask the children to return to their home spots, make a star shape with their bodies, and shine like the word "brillar"!

Modifications

Invite the child to help you call out the Spanish words of the poem while the others move. Quietly prompt her with the words, and then have her repeat them aloud to the group along with you.

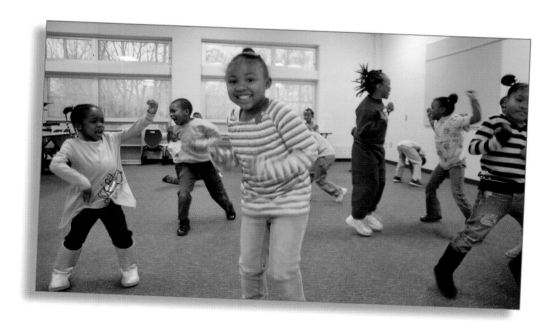

56

Counting Monkeys

• • • • • • • • • • • • • • •

"Counting Monkeys" is a lively activity that addresses the learning of numbers and counting from zero to nine, both forward and backward. The learning is reinforced in several ways: children will listen to the numbers, respond to numbers with corresponding movements, and sing along with the song as they participate in the different portions of the lesson.

What You Need

☼ a small space

☼ "Monkey Fun" (disc 1, track 10)

Explores numbers, shapes, and patterns!

What You Do

Have the children sit in a circle to listen to "Monkey Fun." Say to the children:

We're going to listen to a song and play a game. Pay attention to the lyrics, or words, being sung. The singer will count from zero, or none, up to nine as she sings. "None" means the same thing as zero. Listen carefully, because the singer then says the same numbers again, but this time she counts backward, from nine to none.

Play "Monkey Fun" through several times so the children are familiar with the song and words. While it is playing, prompt the children to count and sing along.

Next each of you will be a number from zero to nine. One or more of the children can have the same number. **We'll listen to the song again, and this time, I want you to stand up when you hear your number. Stay**

standing and listen for the backward counting. When you hear your number sung again, sit down!

Repeat this movement activity many times, letting the children take turns with different numbers to reinforce the learning. To develop the activity, ask the children to think of other movement responses to take the place of standing up and sitting down, and encourage them to count along with the song to reinforce counting skills.

Modifications

Here are some suggestions for other ways to play this game. A child can:

- Make a funny face each time his name is called.
- Make her body into the shape of the number and hold for as long as she can.
- Raise his hands and then lower them when his number is sung in the backward counting.
- Freeze when she hears her number, and then "thaw out" when her number is called in the backward counting.

Encourage the children to create their own movements to go with their numbers when they are called.

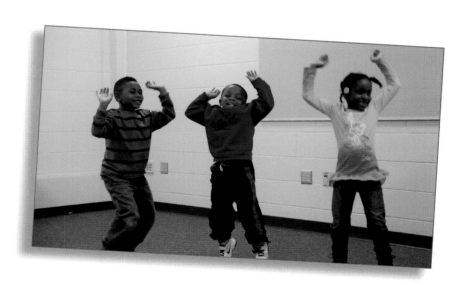

57

Numbers and Patterns

• •

This is a fun and easy way for children to learn about patterns and anticipate the completion of sequences. To continue and expand the activity, use the "Pattern Song" instrumental, make up more patterns, and have the children create their own movement patterns.

What You Need

Explores numbers, shapes, and patterns!

☼ a small space

☼ "Pattern Song" and "Pattern Song" instrumental (disc 1, track 11 and disc 2, track 33)

What You Do

Begin this lesson with the children sitting in a circle. Read the following patterns to the children and ask them to supply the answers at the end:

1, 2; 1, 2; 1, 2; 1, ____

- The children should call out "2."

1, 2, 3; 1, 2, 3; 1, 2, ____

- The children should call out "3."

1, 2, 3, 4; 1, 2, 3, 4; 1, 2, 3, ____

- The children should call out "4."

Next do the same with the pattern words in "Pattern Song." Allow the children to supply the last word in the sequence.

Knees tap, knees tap, knees tap, knees ____

- The children should call out "tap."

Head ear ear, head ear ear, head ear ear, head ____

- The children should call out "ear ear."

Stomp stomp clap, stomp stomp clap, stomp stomp clap, stomp stomp ___

- The children should call out "clap."

Hip hip, zoom zoom; hip hip, zoom zoom; hip hip, zoom zoom; hip hip, ___

- The children should call out "zoom zoom."

Wrist wrist, chin chin chin; wrist wrist, chin chin chin; wrist wrist, chin chin chin; wrist wrist, chin chin ___

- The children should call out "chin."

The next part of the activity can be done with the children sitting in a circle, standing in a circle, or spread about the room in home spots. Put the pattern words together with these movements:

Knees tap

- Tap one knee, then the other.

Head ear ear

- Tap the top of head, one ear, then the other ear.

Stomp stomp clap

- Stomp one foot, the other foot, and then clap hands.

Hip hip zoom zoom

- Touch one hip, then the other hip, and then hold hands on hips and move hips to one side, then to the other side.

Wrist wrist chin chin chin

- Show one wrist, then the other wrist, and then tap chin three times with alternating hands.

Modifications

The children can make up their own movements to go with the patterns. Any movements will work, as long as all the children can do them, and they establish a pattern just as the words in the song do.

Last, put it all together with the music! Play "Pattern Song," and ask the children to first listen and then complete the patterns with words. Play the song again, and do the pattern movements. You can use the instrumental version of the song to continue the activity with your own pattern ideas.

58

One, Two, What Can I Do?

• •

"One, Two, What Can I Do?" is a rhyme with movement suggestions that address counting and numbers. The children learn the poem and respond to the action words while also practicing counting.

What You Need

☼ a small space

Explores numbers, shapes, and patterns!

What You Do

Begin this activity with the children standing in a circle or line, with plenty of room between each child. Position yourself where they can all see you. Explain to the children that they will learn a rhyme and then do movements that go with it. Say the rhyme once, and then repeat it a few times, asking the children to say it along with you.

One, Two, What Can I Do?

Count to one, jump for fun.
One, two, three, I touch my knee.
Four, five, six, quick little kicks.
Seven, eight, nine, my turns are fine.
Now it's ten, let's do it again!

Once the children are familiar with the rhyme, show the movements that go along with each line. Perform the words and movements several times with the children. Start out slowly, and then see how fast you can say the rhyme and do the movements together. Add the last verse when you are ready to finish the activity.

Count to one, jump for fun

- do one big jump on the words "jump for fun"

One, two, three, I touch my knee

- on the words "touch my knee," touch one knee with one hand, then touch the other knee with the other hand, and then touch the first knee with the first hand again

Four, five, six, quick little kicks

- kick with a bent knee, alternating legs three times, on the words "quick little kicks"

Seven, eight, nine, my turns are fine

- turn quickly in place one way, then turn quickly the other way, on the words "my turns are fine"

Now it's ten, let's do it again!

- Repeat the rhyme for as long as the children are engaged. To finish the activity, add this verse:

I count to ten and jump and hop

- jump once, and hop once, on the corresponding words

But now I flop and now I stop!

- flop upper body over

Modifications

Action words in the rhyme can be changed as needed. For example, in the first verse, substitute "bounce" or "stretch" for "jump." In the second line, "bend" or "see" could take the place of "touch." In line three, the little kicks can be performed with arms or fingers instead of legs. In the fourth line, substitute "winks" for "turns," or "my smile is fine" for "my turns are fine." In the sixth line, substitute "shake and bop" for "jump and hop."

59

Move and Freeze

"Move and Freeze" is a good activity to practice listening for cues and following instructions, counting, and reinforcing large-motor skills. In addition, children will learn to understand kinesthetically the concept of motion versus stillness. The freeze game will help the children develop the body control required for stopping and starting.

What You Need

☼ a large space

☼ a drum or a tambourine (optional)

Explores numbers, shapes, and patterns!

What You Do

Ask the children to find a home spot in the room, with plenty of space between them. Say to them:

We're going to play a game about moving and freezing. I'm going to call out a number and a movement to go with the number. I might say "two giant steps," and after you do the two big steps, you'll try to hold very still until I call out the next instruction. If I say "three hops," you'll hop three times and then freeze. What if I say "seven baby steps"? You'll take seven very small steps! I'll count along with you as you do the movements each time, and on each count I'll beat my drum (or tambourine or clap hands).

Here are some more movement suggestions:

- two turns

- one flop to the ground

- four sideways steps

- balance on one foot for five counts

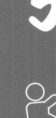

- nine marches

- ten steps on tiptoe

- eight sways from side to side

- three jumps backward

- balance on tiptoe for six counts

- twist your body side to side six times

- four gallops

- throw and catch an imaginary ball in the air two times

- sit down and stand back up four times

- one slow motion fall to the ground

To end the movement activity, ask the children to freeze for ten counts, with everyone counting out loud together. To expand the activity, give each child a turn to think of a number and a movement for everyone to do.

Modifications

Movement can be tailored to the child's own ability when you assign specific movements and when you allow each child to contribute a number and a movement. Ask the child to count out loud with you while the others are responding to the movement instructions.

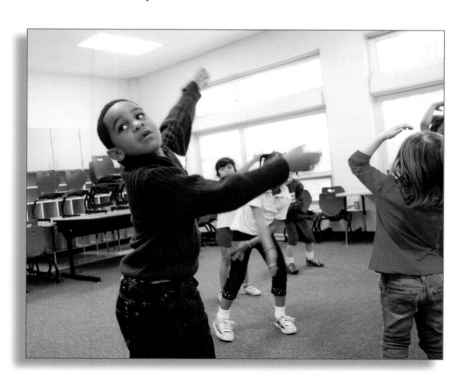

60

Rock the Boat

. . . .

"Rock the Boat" begins as a counting game and develops into an imaginary journey in the ocean. Allow it to evolve as the children's imaginations take them in new directions during the activity. A good follow-up to "Rock the Boat" is Activity 71: Motion in the Ocean.

What You Need

☼ a small space

☼ "Goldie Rock" instrumental (disc 2, track 23)

Explores numbers, shapes, and patterns!

What You Do

Have the children begin by sitting in a circle. Say to them:

Now that we're sitting together in the circle, put the bottoms of your feet together and make your legs into a diamond shape. This is how we make a boat! What would you like to put inside of your boat?

We'll row our boats out into the ocean. Row as fast as you can! Stop and take a rest. Let the waves gently rock your boat. Count to ten with me and sway as we rock from side to side with the waves.

I'd like each of you to choose a number between one and ten. We'll let the waves rock us again, and count along as we sway. When we get to the number you picked, I want you to fall out of your boat! The children should roll gently to their backs or their sides onto the floor when you say their numbers.

We counted all the way to ten, and now we're all in the water! Swim back to your boat. Climb back in. Dry yourself off!

Repeat this several times, asking the children if they would like to choose a different number each time.

Play "Goldie Rock" instrumental and say:

Let's count to ten and fall out of our boats one more time. This time, we'll all fall when we get to ten, and then we'll swim in the ocean to see what we can find! What do you see?

Encourage the children to stand up and imagine they are swimming. Let them dance about the many different things they imagine in the ocean, and play the music again if the children are still engaged. Finish by asking them to swim back to their boats one more time, climb in, dry off, and row back to shore.

Modifications

Allow the child to lead the counting or choose the numbers for the other children as their cues to fall to the floor. Encourage him to participate in the free dance as he is able, responding to the music, the story, and the rhythm in the song.

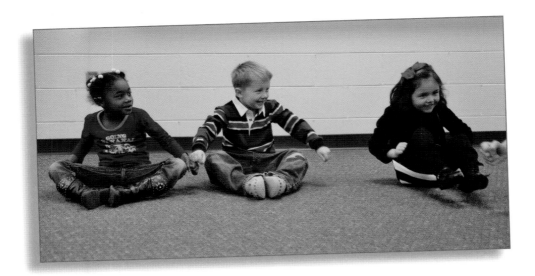

61

Pennies, Nickels, and Dimes

"Pennies, Nickels, and Dimes" is designed for children ages five and up to learn and practice the number value of coins.

What You Need

☼ a small space

☼ a large picture of a penny, a nickel, and a dime

Explores numbers, shapes, and patterns!

What You Do

Place the children side by side in a line, and position yourself so that they all can see you. Say to the children:

A penny is worth one cent, a nickel is worth five cents, and a dime is worth ten cents. I am going to divide you into three groups: one group will be the pennies, one group will be the nickels, and one will be the dimes. Divide the line into three sections, one for each coin.

The pennies will do one big jump each time I show the picture of the penny, because the penny is one cent. The nickels will hop five times each time I show the picture of the nickel. The dimes will run in place for ten counts every time I show the picture of the dime. Count aloud as you do your movement.

Allow each group of children an opportunity to be each coin. For a variation, ask the children to think of new movements for the different coins.

Modifications

The teacher can choose the movements for this game in order to accommodate all the children. For example, if a child has difficulty jumping or hopping, have him put his hands on his hips and flap his arms, or nod his head. Instead of running in place, ask him to clap his hands or tap his feet.

One Plus One Equals Two

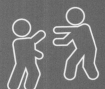

"One Plus One Equals Two" is designed for children ages five and up to use kinesthetic learning to help them understand and reinforce the concept of addition.

What You Need

- ☼ a small space

- ☼ a blackboard or a dry-erase board

Explores numbers, shapes, and patterns!

What You Do

Have the children sit in a circle and say to them:

We are going to do some addition by having our bodies move in different ways! When I call your name, stand up and step just outside the circle. I will give you a movement to do, and tell you how many times to do it. For example, I might say, "Do three skips," or "Do one turn," or "Do four marches."

Once you have done the movements, I'll ask another person to stand up outside the circle to do the same movement a certain number of times. After the second person has performed the movements, both of you will step inside the circle and stand in the center together. Bringing you inside the circle is like joining you together—or like adding two numbers together.

One at a time, each of you will do the movements again. As you do, we'll all count along to figure out the total number of movements you're doing. Then the two of you will return to your home spots, and two more children will try it.

62

For example, you can ask the first child, "Jack," to take a few steps back and do three sways outside the circle. After he does, he should wait there while you ask another child, "Rosa," to step back and do two sways outside the circle. After she does, the two should come inside the circle. Jack then does three sways again, and the group of children counts along. The group continues the count while Rosa does her two sways after Jack.

Use the blackboard or dry-erase board to illustrate the math sentence. Say to the children:

I will make a math sentence out of the movements that Jack and Rosa just did. Three sways, plus two sways, make a total of five sways! Repeat that sentence again with me. Now Jack and Rosa will return to their home spots, and I will ask two more people to take a turn so we can add their movements together and make a new math sentence!

Continue the activity until all the children have had a turn.

Modifications

You can choose appropriate movements for each child. For example, instead of stepping outside the circle, a child may be more comfortable sitting during the activity. Ask her to take just a small scoot back, and give her an upper-body movement, such as two shoulder shrugs, to do. Then ask her to scoot inside the circle to do the shrugs again to complete the math sentence.

From Top to Bottom

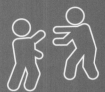

"From Top to Bottom" is designed for children ages five and up to learn, practice, and reinforce the correct way to write numbers. It can also be done to recharge the children's energy and focus during writing practice, allowing them a quick break between small-motor skill exercises.

Explores numbers, shapes, and patterns!

What You Need

☼ a small space (the free dance at the end of the activity can be done moving throughout the shared space)

☼ "Monkey Fun" (disc 1, track 10)

☼ a large card or picture showing each number, one through nine

What You Do

Ask the children to stand in a circle with plenty of space between them. Say to the children:

We are going to practice writing numbers today, but we are going to write them in the air! Let's all pick up our magic pencils. Look at the picture of the number "1." I am going to take my magic pencil and draw the number "1" in the air. I start at the top, and then make a straight line in the air. Let's all try that! Now instead of our pencils, let's draw the number "1" with our noses! Start at the top, just as you did before.

Guide the children to write the number "1" in the air using the nose, then foot, shoulder, wrist, head, knee, hip, and chin, while staying in their home spots. Continue this exercise until the children have practiced writing all of the numbers from one to nine.

To expand this activity, play "Monkey Fun" and allow the children to practice all the letters in a free dance, either in place or around the room. Say:

Modifications

A child may do the entire lesson (using the imaginary pencil, leading with body parts to write the numbers, and moving freely) either sitting or lying down while the others are moving about the space. He can hold up the number cards for you as you introduce each new number, and you can invite him to sing along with the words in the song.

During this free dance, you can write numbers with your magic pencil, write the numbers in the air using different parts of the body, or just dance to the music. Listen for the numbers in the song!

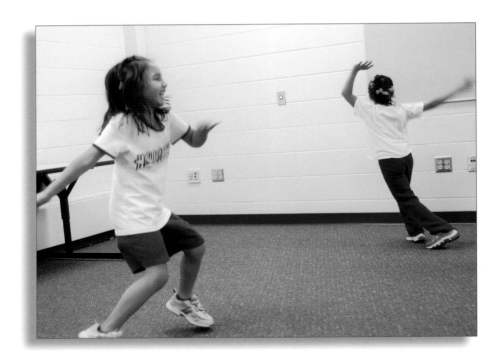

Muscle Mania

· · · · · · · · · · ·

"Muscle Mania" introduces children to the correct way to warm up before participating in more strenuous activities—and helps establish lifelong healthy exercise habits! This is a good follow-up to Activity 12: Wake Up, Muscles.

What You Need

Explores science!

☼ a large space

☼ "Stronger" instrumental (disc 2, track 41)

What You Do

Say to the children:

Today we're going to learn how our muscles help make our body parts move! Doing these exercises can also make our muscles strong. Our muscles work best when we warm them up, first with slow movements and then working up to bigger and faster movements. We'll learn some fun warm-ups you can do before you exercise, or anytime!

Let's begin by sitting in a circle, with our legs crossed and sitting up very straight. Our stomach and back muscles help keep us sitting tall.

Your face has many moving parts! Can you move your forehead and eyebrows up and down? Can you move just your eyes? Look side to side, up and down. Make your eyes wide and then squint. Open and close them a few times. Can you open one eye and close the other? Now switch eyes. Can you wink? A wink is a gesture that says "hello!"

Now open your mouth very wide. Close it. The muscles in your jaw are helping move your mouth so you can eat, talk, smile, and frown. Did you know it takes many more muscles to frown than to smile? Let's practice smiling and frowning. Now stick your tongue out, wiggle it around, and bring it back in. Can you do that again? Let's finish the mouth movements by saying "hello" to the people next to us.

It's mostly the muscles in your neck that move your head, and your head can move in many directions. Try nodding your head, like saying "yes," and then try shaking it from side to side, like saying "no." Now turn your head even farther to the side and then to the other side. Repeat that several times. Look way up to the ceiling and then down to the floor. Put your ear close to your shoulder and then do that with your other ear.

Lift your shoulders high and then bring them down. Do that several times. Shrugging our shoulders is how we say "I don't know," isn't it? Can you move your shoulders up and down one at a time, then together? Now move them together forward and back, then in a circle coming forward first, and then back. Can you alternate your shoulders' circling, first one, and then the other, several times?

Squeeze your hands into tight fists and then open them up. Let's do that a few more times. Wiggle your fingers slowly, then quickly. Can you circle your hands from your wrists? Wave to someone across the circle, first with one hand, then the other, then with both hands. Now shake out your hands and fingers.

Put your hands on your shoulders, so your arms look like wings. Flap your wings! Now circle your shoulders so your wings make big circles, and repeat the circles the other way. Take your arms straight up and let them drop down, and repeat that a few times. Take your arms out to the side, and then wrap them around and give yourself a big hug!

Now we'll move the whole upper body, or torso, using some big muscles. Put one hand on the floor next to you, and let your whole upper body bend to that side, reaching your other arm over as far as you can.

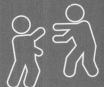

Now go back up to the center, where you started, and try the bending and reaching to the other side, and finish by coming back to the center again.

Put your hands on your knees and look at the ceiling—let your chest reach up to the ceiling too. Next put your hands on the floor in front of you and gently flop forward. Come back up. Can you twist your torso around to one side so you can look behind you? Now do the same thing on the other side. Finish by making a circle with your upper body: move to the side, forward, side, up, and then the other way.

Let's stand up in our home spots. Can you scrunch your toes and then let them relax? Take your arms out to the side to help you balance, and try picking up one leg. Wiggle your toes, and then use your ankle muscles to move your raised foot around in many different directions. Can you make a circle with your foot? Wave to someone with your foot! Repeat with the other foot.

Stand on both feet and, using your arms for balance again, bend both your knees and straighten them several times. Now bend them and go all the way up to your toes. Can you balance on your tiptoes for a few seconds? Come back down.

Lift one leg and see how many ways you can move it while you balance on the other leg. Do the same with the other side. Let's shake out our legs one at a time. Now we'll finish our exercises by shaking our whole bodies out while we stay in our home spots. Shake for ten counts, and freeze at the end when I clap.

Now that we've warmed up the muscles in all the different parts of our bodies, let's use them all together!

I'll play the music. While it's playing, I'd like you to move around the room, watching out for the other children. Use any of the movements we've done today, and think about other ways you like to move using your muscles!

64

Play "Stronger" instrumental and let the children dance freely until the music ends. Play the instrumental again if the children need more time. The following are a few optional prompts:

- **Can you take big steps as you walk?**

- **Try walking high on your tiptoes, using your foot and leg muscles, and reaching your arms to the ceiling.**

- **Can you walk fast?**

- **Can you turn?**

- **Can you hop? On the other foot?**

- **Can you jump while you're moving around?**

- **Can you shake?**

Modifications

Ask children to lead different parts of the warm-up according to their abilities. For example, if a child has difficulty standing, call on her to show one of the upper-body warm-ups: "Watch how Mary can circle her arms! Let's try to do it like Mary!" Another child who uses a wheelchair can lead the head and neck movements: "Can you nod your head like Joey? Now let's move our heads up and down and side to side like he does!"

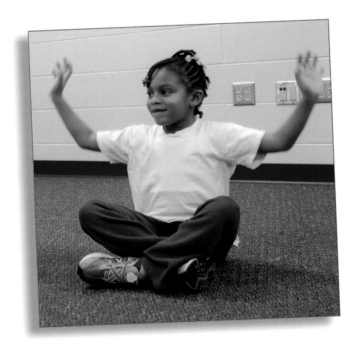

Imagine

This poem is filled with vivid images about the natural world. The descriptive words will inspire the children's imaginations and spur creative movement ideas.

What You Need

Explores science!

☼ a large space, indoors or outside

☼ "Care of the Earth" instrumental (disc 1, track 16)

What You Do

Ask the children to go to home spots spread throughout the large space. Read the poem aloud to them one time through.

Imagine

Light as a feather you begin to fly
Through cottony clouds way up in the sky.
You soar and float, you dive and dip,
Catch the wind, turn and flip.

Or tumble like water in a chilly creek
All the way down from a mountain peak.
Turn and laugh, sparkle and flash,
Through hills and valleys, you jump and splash.

A tiny seed hiding under the ground,
You sprout and grow, your vines wind round.
Higher and higher, you climb and spread
Until flowers burst forth, shiny and red.

Say to the children:

This poem has three parts, or verses, and each one describes movement inspired by the natural world. I will read the first verse again.

Light as a feather you begin to fly
Through cottony clouds way up in the sky.
You soar and float, you dive and dip,
Catch the wind, turn and flip.

What do you think the first verse is about? Flying—that's right! Let's try some flying ourselves. I will put on some music, and you will dance about flying. You may move around the space, but remember to watch out for the other children. Think about being light as a feather in the sky, and soar, float, dive, dip. Feel the wind, imagine the clouds. Come in for a slow, steady landing, and end up on your home spot.

Play "Care of the Earth" instrumental. Turn off the music when the children have arrived back in their home spots.

Now, let's do the same thing with the second verse. Listen carefully as I read it.

Or tumble like water in a chilly creek
All the way down from a mountain peak.
Turn and laugh, sparkle and flash,
Through hills and valleys, you jump and splash.

What would it be like to be a flowing creek, tumbling down a mountain? I will start the music again, and we will turn, laugh, sparkle, and flash. Let's finish in our home spots, after flowing all the way down the tall mountain.

Turn the music off when the children have finished exploring these movement ideas.

The third verse is about something that grows, which is a different kind of movement. I will read the third verse again.

**A tiny seed hiding under the ground,
You sprout and grow, your vines wind round.
Higher and higher, you climb and spread
Until flowers burst forth, shiny and red.**

**Now imagine you are a seed. What kind of seed would you like to be?
Hide underground, and when I start the music, you can begin to grow.**

Allow the children to explore this idea, and then tell them to try to hold
their plant shape for a few seconds once you turn the music off.

**To finish, I will play the music one more time, all the way through. This
time you can dance freely throughout the space about all three verses
of the poem, thinking about flying, bubbling
like a creek, and growing very tall like a
plant. When the music is finished, make a
final shape about flying through the sky.**

Modifications

Invite the child to help you call out the words
of the poem while the others move. Quietly
prompt her with the words to each line, and
then invite her to call them out to the group
with you. Bring in pictures of different flying
animals (birds, bats, butterflies), mountains
and streams, and different kinds of plants, so
the child can hold them up during the corresponding part of the activity.

66

Dance Story—
Baby Birdie Boogie

• • • • • • • • • • • • • •

"Baby Birdie Boogie" contains a series of movement images centered on the tale of a baby bird who hatches out of an egg and learns to fly! This activity ends with a free dance, which allows the children to use their imaginations to explore all the ideas presented in the activity.

What You Need

Explores science!

☼ a large space

☼ "Little Birdie" and "Little Birdie" instrumental (disc 1, track 9 and disc 2, track 29)

What You Do

Designate a home spot for each child somewhere in the shared dancing space so each has a nest to return to during and at the end of the dance. Play "Little Birdie" instrumental quietly in the background. Say to the children:

Can you imagine what it would be like to be a baby bird? Baby birds begin their lives as eggs in a warm nest. Find a place in the room, in the open space, that you can imagine as your nest. Curl up inside your egg. It's not time for you to come out yet! What does it feel like while you are waiting?

Now it's time for the baby birds to come into the world. Use your tiny beak to peck at the inside of the shell of the egg. It's hard! Keep pecking until you peck through the shell. Now take your little foot and try to push through the egg. Push and push! Push with your other leg. Now try pushing with one wing and then the other! Peck some more, and pretty soon, look—you've come out of your shell.

Baby birds are hungry! Let's imagine that our mama bird is going to bring us some food. Yum, yum: worms! Open your birdie mouths! Say "thank you." What soft sounds do baby birds make?

Just as you had to learn to walk as a baby, baby birds have to learn to fly. Let's try out our wings first. Slowly flap your little wings. As they get stronger and you get bigger, you can flap them harder.

Now it's time to leave the nest. Stand at the edge and look down—it's a long way down, because you are high up in a tree. Ready, set, try to fly. Uh-oh, you're falling! Flap those wings, fast, faster, as fast as you can! Look, you're flying, baby birds! Fly all around the room, and look around you as you fly. What do you see up high in the sky? Fly back to your nest (the home spot) **and rest after your first day of learning to fly.**

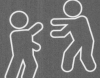

To continue this activity, delineate a space in the room where you can all sit comfortably in a group. This will be the nest for all of the baby birds to sit in at once. If there are a large number of children, you can divide them into two groups, with one group watching while the other is dancing. Give a task to the group that is watching; for example, ask them "What else might be flying in the sky with the birdies?"

Play "Little Birdie." Ask the children to come together to the nest, and tell them it's time to practice flying. Sit in the nest while the children fly around the room, and then call the baby birds back one by one. Repeat this several times.

Modifications

A child who is unable to participate in the larger movement portions of this activity can sit in the nest and call the birds back one by one. You can bring or make a series of pictures of the different stages of a bird's development as it is told throughout the story: egg, hatching, baby bird sitting in the nest, eating, and flying. The child can hold up the different pictures as they correspond to the story while the other children do the movement. An additional way for children to participate is to sing along with the words in the song.

Continue to play the music and finish with a free dance. Encourage the children to use ideas from the activity: a baby bird waiting in an egg, emerging from the egg, learning to fly, leaving and then coming back to the nest. Prompt the children to respond to the many movement images in the song: "Fly up high, fly down low, fly real slow, take a rest in the nest." Finish with all the baby birds flying back into the nest, to take a rest, just like in the song.

I Can

Vivid movement images from the animal kingdom in this poem serve as prompts for the children to explore many different locomotor skills and movement qualities. The free dance reinforces the practicing of the skills and provides an opportunity for further exploration of the poem's images. "I Can" will really get children moving!

What You Need

Explores science!

☼ a large space, indoors or outside

☼ "Cygnet" instrumental (disc 1, track 19)

What You Do

Ask the children to stand in a line spread out across one end of the large space, and read the poem through one time.

I Can

I can bounce like a bunny.
I can pounce like a cat.
I can slither like a snake.
Fly zigzag like a bat.

I can run like a deer.
I can jump like a frog.
I can crawl like a crab.
Wag my tail like a dog.

I can dart like a fish.
I can dive like a whale.
I can gallop like a deer.
Crawl slowly like a snail.

I can bend, turn, and twist.
I can jump very high.
I can do so many things.
All I have to do is try!

Now the children will respond in movement, one by one, to the first fourteen lines of the poem. (If there are more than fourteen children in the group, have two children respond to some of the lines together.) For example, the first child will respond to the first line, "I can bounce like a bunny," by hopping all the way to the other side of the space. The second child moves to the second line, "I can pounce like a cat," to the other side of the space, joining the first child, and so on.

Once every child has had a turn to dance a line of the poem, tell the children to get ready to go back across the floor together. Read each line of the poem again. This time the children will respond together to each line, moving across the floor as they "bounce like a bunny," and then back across as they "pounce like a cat," and so on.

All together the children will move back and forth across the floor until the last two lines of the poem: "I can do so many things" and "All I have to do is try!" Invite the children to go across together one last time when you say these last two lines aloud, doing any—or many—of the movements from the poem.

Finish the activity with a free dance. Ask the children to spread out in the space and find a home spot. Remind them of the many images in the poem. Play "Cygnet" instrumental and prompt them to dance freely in the large space using any and all of the movement ideas. At the music's end, have the children return to their home spots and freeze in the shape of one of the animals mentioned in the poem.

Modifications

Invite the child to help you call out the words of the poem while the others are moving. Quietly prompt her with the words, and then have her repeat them aloud to the group along with you. You can also bring in pictures of the various animals mentioned in the poem, and ask the child to hold them up as you say the corresponding lines in the poem.

68

Dance Story— Dinosaur Romp

• • • • • • • • • • • • • •

"Dinosaur Romp" is a lively movement activity. Use this dance story as a prompt for the children, pacing it so that the movements can unfold and develop. The story and song have many references to dinosaurs, their qualities and habitats. The second part of this activity allows children to dance freely to the music, reinforcing ideas from the dance story.

Explores science!

What You Need

☼ a large space, indoors or outside (if you have only a small space, each child can move within a home spot, and a large group of children can be divided into smaller groups)

☼ "Dinosaur Romp" (disc 1, track 2)

What You Do

Ask the children to go to their home spots, spread throughout the shared space. If you divide the children into groups, try to engage the group that is watching by giving the children a prompt, such as, "What else do you think you would see if you could go back to the time of the dinosaurs? Can you think of other dinosaurs you might find?" Say to the children:

Wouldn't it be fun if we could see a dinosaur? Dinosaurs lived in the past, so we'll try to imagine what it would be like to take a trip to visit dinosaurs.

Let's put on our dinosaur-watching gear. First put on your swamp pants and your jacket. Pull on your big boots. Get your hat. Get your binoculars and your map! What else do we need? The most important thing we need is our imaginations. Let's turn them on! Here we go!

Squish slowly through the swamp. It's difficult to walk in the swamp, with all this mud! Your feet are getting stuck, so pull hard to keep walking. Now you can't get them out at all, but keep trying! What will you do? Quick, reach for that branch. Hang on to the branch. Pull your feet out as hard as you can. Swing across that big puddle. Jump down from the branch. Look, here comes a brontosaurus! Isn't he big? His footsteps are so heavy and loud! Let's stomp like the brontosaurus.

Now look, the brontosaurus is stomping away—but here comes a pterodactyl! The pterodactyl was a prehistoric reptile that could fly. Let's imagine we're all pterodactyls. Take off from the ground. Fly out of the swamp! Fly far over the mountains, over the water. What do you see? Do you know which other dinosaurs lived a long time ago? Do you see any of them far down below? Flap your giant wings as fast as you can! Now come in for a landing.

We've landed, but look! Here is another dinosaur. A tyrannosaurus—look how big he is! His teeth are also big and he is chomping. Can you chomp like that?

Now it's time to go. Sneak away from the swamp. Let's be quiet so the dinosaurs don't see us! Walk quickly back to your home spots. Put away your dinosaur-watching gear. What a fun adventure!

Now I'll put on a song called "Dinosaur Romp," which is about the imaginary adventure we just took. I'm going to play it, and you can move to the music, dancing freely in the large space. When you move, you can go on another adventure, you can listen to the lyrics and dance about some of the action words you hear—"stomp," "flap," "squish," "sneak," "fly"—and you can feel the beat of the music and have fun! When the music stops, go to your home spot and make yourself into the shape of your favorite kind of dinosaur.

Modifications

A suggestion to include the child who is unable to participate in the movements in this lesson is to bring or make a series of pictures of the three prehistoric creatures explored in the story and song: brontosaurus, pterodactyl, and tyrannosaurus. The child can hold up the different pictures as they correspond to the story while the other children are doing the corresponding movement. An additional way for children to participate is to sing along with the words in the song.

69

I Love to Move

The children will celebrate their bodies and all the ways their bodies can move, as they dance to this playful poem. They will learn new words along the way, such as "sturdy" and "steady"!

What You Need

☼ a small space

☼ "Happy Face" (disc 1, track 6)

Explores science!

What You Do

Ask the children to sit in a circle or in home spots throughout the room. Begin by reading the poem aloud one time.

I Love to Move

My smile is cheerful and bright.
My eyes are shiny and clear.
My bones are big and sturdy.
My two ears help me hear.

My lungs have a regular rhythm
As they breathe air in and out.
My heartbeat is soft and steady.
My strong voice likes to shout!

My muscles help me move.
I love to learn and play.
So many different things
To do throughout the day!

Now read the poem again and slowly go through the movements with the children.

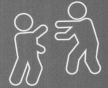

My smile is cheerful and bright.

- point to your mouth, smile, and draw a smile in the air

My eyes are shiny and clear.

- point to your eyes, and draw two eyes in the air

My bones are big and sturdy.

- touch your arms, legs, head, torso, feet, hands

My two ears help me hear.

- point to your ears, and draw two ears in the air

My lungs have a regular rhythm

- place your hands on your ribs

As they breathe air in and out.

- feel your lungs rise and fall as you breathe

My heartbeat is soft and steady.

- place your hands on your chest and feel your heartbeat

My strong voice likes to shout!

- signal "1, 2, 3" with your fingers and then shout, covering your ears; hold up your hand to signal the end of the shout

My muscles help me move.

- stand up in your home spot

I love to learn and play.

- move as many ways as you can: bend and twist and turn

So many different things

- jump and hop

To do throughout the day!

- go down to the floor and back up to standing

Repeat the poem and movements together a couple of times, until the children know the movement responses. Encourage them to say the words along with you as they become familiar with them. To continue the activity, say to the children:

Now I will put on the song "Happy Face." You may move from your spot and dance freely. Dance about the different parts of the body described in the poem, the ones we pointed to and drew in the air, and about all the different ways our bones and muscles help us move!

When the music ends, say to the children:

Let's go back to our home spots. Now put your hands on your ribs again, and feel your lungs. You are breathing hard after all that dancing! That is good! It makes your lungs stronger. Now place your hands on your chest. Your heart is beating fast and getting stronger from the all exercise you did!

Modifications

A child may be able to do many of the movements while sitting or lying down. Invite the child to help you call out the words of the poem while the others move. Quietly prompt her with the words to each line, and then invite her to call them out to the group with you. Bring pictures of different body parts for the child to hold up as you name them.

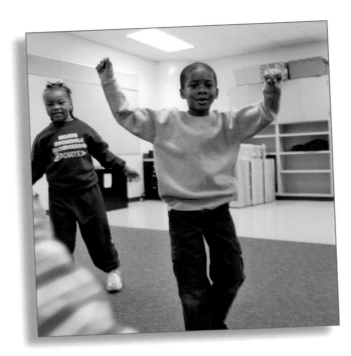

Eating Healthy

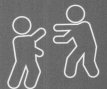

"Eating Healthy" is a movement exploration made up of three activities that can be taught together or individually. Each is a kinesthetic approach to helping children understand how food can affect how they feel. This helps the children learn about making healthy food choices.

Explores science!

What You Need

☆ a large space

☆ "Eating Healthy" and "Catsup" instrumental (disc 1, tracks 3 and 17)

☆ a collage of healthy foods, a collage of junk foods, and pom-poms for the children

Tired or Energetic?

What You Do

Begin with the children standing in a circle with plenty of room between them. Ask them to practice falling gently to their seats, catching themselves with their hands so they don't get hurt. Bring them back to standing, and then say to them:

Let's start by thinking about two different feelings: tired and energetic. Staying in your home spots, go down to the floor as if you were so tired you couldn't stand up any longer. Now stand up with lots of energy! Oh, no. . . . Your energy is gone again, and this time, you're so tired you have to move in slow motion. Now stand up the same way—in slow motion. This time, sit down with lots of energy! Remember to catch yourselves with your hands.

We usually move in a lively way when we have lots of energy, and we usually move slowly and feel sleepy and heavy when we don't. Did you feel the difference?

Continue this game by mixing the movement ideas: up and down, fast and slow, tired and energetic. Finish the activity with everyone standing.

Feel the Fuel

What You Do

The children should be standing in a circle, with plenty of space between them. Say to them:

Do you know the foods we eat can make us feel tired or energetic? Let's think about how fuel works in a car: bad fuel makes the car sputter and stop, and good fuel keeps the car going steady and strong. Let's try that! Imagine you're a car, and somebody just put bad fuel in you. Turn away from the circle and walk slowly as you sputter and stop, and sputter and stop, just like a car that's breaking down. Now turn around and come back to your home spot like a car with good fuel in its tank!

Now let's try it as if we were rocket ships. Let's crouch low and see what happens with bad fuel. Uh-oh! We can't get off the ground! We try, but we just can't do it. Now we have good fuel in our rocket ships. Let's crouch down and count from ten down to one together: 10, 9, 8, 7, 6, 5, 4, 3, 2, 1, blast off! Everyone jump high up into the air!

Be a Healthy-Eating Hero and Not a Junk Food Dude

What You Do

Two simple visual cues—made by you or by the children—can enhance this movement game: a collage or drawing of the Healthy-Eating Hero (a human shape made up of pictures of vegetables, fruits, grains, and lean meats) and a collage or drawing of Junk Food Dude (a human shape made

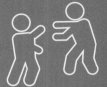

of pictures of doughnuts, candy, soda, and other unhealthy items). The children should be standing in their home spots throughout the shared space. Hold up the two collages and say:

Look at the food the Junk Food Dude likes to eat. Now look at the food the Healthy-Eating Hero eats. Junk foods and healthy foods both provide fuel for our bodies, just like gas is fuel for a car or a rocket ship, but one type of food is a better fuel for your body and gives you better energy. Can you guess which one? Let's think of some foods that are healthy, and some that are not.

We'll show this idea in movement. When I hold up the picture of the Junk Food Dude, you walk around slowly in a small circle, as if you were very tired. When I hold up the picture of the Healthy-Eating Hero, you march, hop, or jump! Stay in your home spot while we do these movements; that way we don't have to worry about bumping into each other. Proceed to hold up one collage, and then the other, and repeat this exercise a few times.

Next we'll try this game moving around to music. When I hold up the Healthy-Eating Hero, I'll play some fast music. Play "Catsup" instrumental. **When you hear this music, do the energetic movements—march, hop, or jump—as you travel around the room. I won't play the music when I hold up the Junk Food Dude, and the only movement you can do when you see the Junk Food Dude is to walk in slow motion in a small circle.**

When the song ends, ask the children which way of moving they prefer.

Let's finish with two free dances about the importance of eating healthy. This music, "Eating Healthy," has a strong marching beat to it, so let's start by listening to the music, staying in one spot, and clapping the rhythm. Listen carefully to the words in the song about eating good, healthy foods. Play "Eating Healthy."

Can you hear the steady beat? Let's keep the rhythm using our legs and feet, stepping with each beat in the music. Now march around the room. Pick up those knees! Can you point your toes when your feet are in the air? Stop and keep the beat with your arms, swinging them like you do when you march, then march with your feet and your arms

together. Now clap your hands while you march. Can you march low? Can you march on your tiptoes with your arms high in the air? Freeze when the music stops!

Pass out the pom-poms and give one or two to each child to hold and shake with their hands. Play "Eating Healthy" one more time.

We'll do one more free dance to this song, using a fun prop! While you're dancing, think about the things we've learned about eating healthy: some foods leave us feeling tired, and some foods make us feel energetic; bad fuel and good fuel; and the Healthy-Eating Hero and the Junk Food Dude. You can also practice the many different ways that we marched, holding and shaking the pom-poms while you march.

Finish the dance with each person freezing in the shape of a fruit or a vegetable.

Modifications

Bring pictures of cars and rocket ships and ask a child to hold them up while others are dancing about cars and then rocket ships. Ask the child if he would like to make car and rocket ship sounds with his voice. He could also lead the counting in the rocket ship activity.

During "Be a Healthy-Eating Hero and Not a Junk Food Dude," give the child the task of holding up the collage props. During the last part of the activity, give him pom-poms to hold and manipulate while the other children use them in the free dance. An additional way for children to participate is to sing along with the words in the song "Eating Healthy."

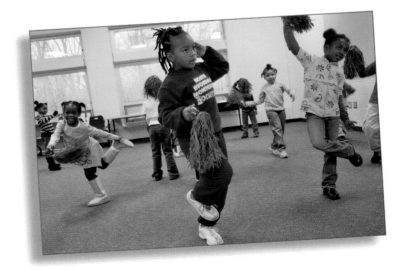

Motion in the Ocean

A poem about undersea exploration sets the stage for a lively movement activity that will spark the imagination. The descriptions of marine animals and images of the sea will elicit many creative responses from the children.

Explores science!

What You Need

☼ a large space

☼ "Goldie Waltz" instrumental and "Goldie Rock" instrumental (disc 2, tracks 24 and 23)

☼ colorful crepe paper or fabric streamers (no longer than twelve inches)

What You Do

Begin with the children seated in a circle. Say to them:

Today we're going to go on a deep sea exploration! What do you think we will see? First I have a poem to read to you, and then we'll dance the poem.

Motion in the Ocean

**Let's go exploring down under the ocean
To see all the wonderful creatures in motion!**

**Let's dive down deep, still deeper we go
It's sparkly and blue where the cool waters flow.**

**See the strange squid and the octopi
Waving and swirling as we go by.**

**See the smooth dolphins, seals, and whales
Gliding and jumping and flapping their tails.**

**Look at the schools of colorful fish
Darting and turning as their fins go swish.**

**Look at the sea horses upright and proud
Listen real close, do they whinny out loud?**

**Now float to the surface and look at the sky
See seagulls and pelicans gracefully fly!**

**Waves push you gently now back to the shore
Hear far in the distance the ocean's loud roar.**

**You can go to the ocean anytime that you wish
To visit the lobsters and oysters and fish.**

**Imagine you're back in the deep, deep blue ocean
To dance to the rhythm of the waves in motion!**

Ask the children to go to a home spot in the room while you play "Goldie Waltz" softly in the background. Say to the children:

Let's put on our scuba-diving gear! First we'll put on our wet suits, then our fins, and then our masks. Is everyone ready? Let's take a big jump on our home spots and go down into the ocean.

Now read the poem again, slowly. Pause after each line so the children can respond in movement, moving freely throughout the space. Play the music over as many times as needed so you have a musical background through-out the reading and while the children dance.

When you are ready to begin the next part of the activity, say to the children:

Now we're going to dance about the poem one more time. I'll pass out these streamers, which will help us imagine the waves and the many soft, swaying plants and animals in the water. I'll put on some different music too. As you dance, think about the poem and about moving many

different ways with the streamer. You can also dance about any other ideas you have about the sea! Play "Goldie Rock" instrumental.

Finish the activity by asking the children to make a final shape while holding their streamers. A couple of possible prompts are:

- **Can you make a shape like seaweed, with its many branches?**

- **What shape would you make if you were a curvy little eel?**

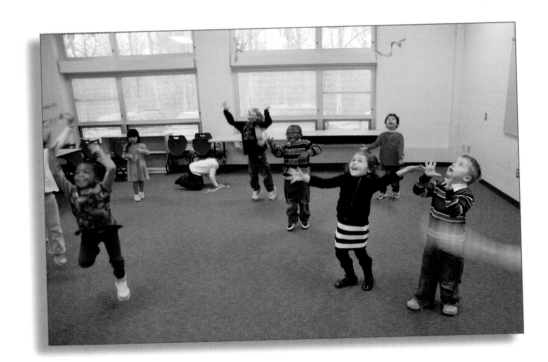

Modifications

Invite the child to help you call out the words of the poem while the others are moving. Quietly prompt him with the words before you say each line, and then have him repeat them aloud to the group with you. Give the child a streamer to hold and manipulate in response to the poem and music, so he can be included in the activity.

72

Dance Story— Monkey Movin'
• • • • • • • • • •

There are many ideas about monkeys in this musical activity, including their behavior, movements, and habitat. Use the song "Monkey Fun" as a prompt to inspire the children as the movements unfold and develop. The second part of this movement activity allows children to dance freely to the music, reinforcing ideas from the dance story.

Explores science!

What You Need

☼ a large space (if you have only a small space, each child can move within a home spot, and a large group of children can be divided into smaller groups)

☼ "Monkey Fun" (disc 1, track 10)

What You Do

Ask the children to go to home spots spread throughout the shared space. If you divide the children into groups, try to engage the group that is watching by giving the children a prompt, such as, "Have you seen monkeys in the zoo? What did they do? Did they climb and swing from their tails? Watch the other children, and see what they do!" Say to the children:

Let's imagine this room is a jungle. Look at all the trees! Monkeys like to climb and play in trees, so everyone find a tree to climb. First reach your arms around the tree to see how big it is. Now, climb! Up, up, up! Look, we're high above the jungle! What can you see? Are there other animals that like to be high up in the trees?

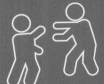

Monkeys get a lot of exercise. Use your long arms to help you get up and down the tree. First let's climb slowly down the tree, and then let's climb slowly back up. Let's climb down again, a little faster, and then up one more time as fast as we can! Finish by standing on the very top branch of your tree. Wave to all the other monkeys at the tops of their trees! Say a "How de do" to them!

Do you feel hungry? Reach for some fruit. Yum! Taste it! It's sweet and juicy. There's fruit all over your tree. Let's gather some! Now let's climb back down.

Let's try some of the action words in the song we're going to listen to. We already did some climbing, which is an action word in the song, so let's try jumping. Jump in place and then around the room—watch out for the other monkeys! Now let's try skating. Put on your monkey roller skates and skate around the room.

What tricks can monkeys do? Use your imagination and try some monkey tricks. Let's try some jiving and dancing—just do whatever you want to do—and then we'll try all of the movements with music.

Play "Monkey Fun" and let the children respond to the words of the music as they wish.

Remember all the action words we talked about today? You can dance about any of those, and also use your imaginations to dance about any of our ideas about monkeys or other animals in the jungle—whatever you wish! The song finishes with "taking a seat," which would be a good ending for our activity. How would a great big monkey get down to the floor? Take a seat and feel the beat!

Modifications

To include all children in this activity's movements, bring or make a series of pictures of monkeys doing the various things mentioned: climbing, eating, jumping, skating, and so on. A child can hold up the different pictures as they correspond to the story and movement. The child can also sing the song and make monkey noises while the other children dance!

73

Parade
• • • • • • •

The movements in "Parade" correspond to the festive sounds in the "Marching Band" instrumental. This is a fun activity to use to commemorate Memorial Day, Veterans Day, Presidents' Day, or the Fourth of July, and the children will enjoy hearing the rhythm and marching to the beat in the music.

Explores social studies!

What You Need

☼ a large space, indoors or outside

☼ "Marching Band" instrumental (disc 2, track 30)

☼ small American flags or red, white, and blue fabric or crepe-paper streamers (no longer than twelve inches)

What You Do

To begin, ask the children to stand in their home spots spread throughout the shared space. The children will dance in their home spots, move freely in the shared space, and line up to form a parade. During the parade, the children will take turns being the leader. Say to them:

I'll play the music, and I'd like you to listen to the beat. Play "Marching Band" instrumental. **Let's all try clapping to the beat while we're listening. Now try to feel that strong beat in your feet, and let's march in place to the beat. Pick up those knees! Now try clapping and marching in place at the same time!**

Pass out a prop to each child. Play "Marching Band" instrumental again and encourage the children to move freely to the music throughout the shared space. While they are moving, challenge them to do the following movement tasks:

- **Keep marching to the music's strong beat, and lift your knees high into the air!**

- **March in a small circle in your home spot. Now try it turning around the other way. Can you march quietly? Now stomp your feet!**

- **Let's hold onto our props and line up behind "Amanda." She'll be our first leader, and then everyone else will take a turn leading our parade.**

- **Now I'll play the music again, and you march freely throughout the shared space again. Try using the props in different ways—shake them, twirl them, move them high and then low, jump with them, and toss them up in the air and catch them.**

Modifications

Instead of marching, a child can clap to the beat or move another part of the body, such as the head or foot, in time to the music. In addition, he can manipulate the prop during that section of the lesson. He can also hold up pictures that represent the holiday you might be commemorating—for example, pictures of a flag, fireworks, and a parade for the Fourth of July.

To end the activity, say to the children:

Let's finish our activity by marching back to our home spots. I'll come around and collect the props. That was a lot of marching! Sit down in your spot, and let's take a rest!

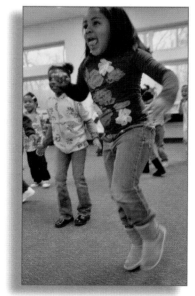

Dance Story—
Digging the Dirt

"Digging the Dirt" gives children the opportunity to dance the movements of creating a garden: digging, planting, caring for and harvesting the plants. It allows the children to use their imaginations while learning about a plant's growth from seed to fruit, as well as how to tend a garden.

What You Need

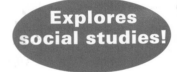

Explores social studies!

☼ a large space

☼ "Dig, Dig, Dig" (disc 1, track 1)

☼ pictures of community gardens

What You Do

If you have access to it, use a space big enough for all the children to be included at once. Delineate a square in the space by showing children the imaginary garden area, or, if you prefer, create the space using a rug, mats, or a border made of chairs, where you'll plant the garden. Bring the children together in the garden space and ask them to sit down. Show them pictures of community gardens—or ask the children to draw some in conjunction with this activity—and say to them:

Today we're going to dance about planting a garden together! Here are some pictures of community gardens, where people work together to plant beautiful flowers and healthy foods. What kinds of flowers and foods do you think people plant in community gardens? This large space where we're sitting is where we'll plant our community garden. Your spot within this space is where you'll work on the garden.

Play "Dig, Dig, Dig." Say to the children:

What's the first thing we should do? Dig the dirt! Everybody stand up and get your shovels and start digging! Now we'll plant the seeds, just like the song says. Take your seeds and plant them down low! Make sure they're tucked into the soil. Now cover them up with soil. What kinds of seeds are you planting? Won't it be fun to see them start to grow?

Next we must water them. Get your watering cans and give them some water. Here they come—our plants are growing! But we must weed them so they have lots of room to grow and spread. Take your hoe and dig out those weeds, and pull them out with your hands too.

Our plants are big and beautiful now. Let's harvest them before it gets cold. Let's each take a great big basket and pick our flowers and vegetables! Our baskets are heavy. Can you carry such a heavy basket? Isn't it amazing that we grew all of these lovely flowers and vegetables ourselves?

Be sure to allow time for the children to develop each movement in response to the prompt. Repeat the song while there is still interest in the activity.

Modifications

A child can sit in the garden space and respond to whatever parts of the dance story she can. She can also hold up pictures of the different stages of gardens during the dance story, and pictures of different fruits, vegetables, and flowers to be found in a community garden.

75

Grocery Space Trip

The song "Grocery Space Trip" is rich in images and movement prompts, and perfect for exploring ideas through three mediums: drawing, music, and dancing. This is a good follow-up to Activity 24: Space Suits.

What You Need

Explores social studies!

☼ a large space

☼ "Grocery Space Trip" (disc 1, track 5)

☼ crayons and drawing paper

What You Do

Pass out paper and crayons and play "Grocery Space Trip." Ask the children to draw something based on images they hear in the song. Play the song a few times while the children work on their drawings.

Ask the children to put their papers aside and go to their home spots, ready to dance. Explain that they can dance about what they drew and other parts of the song. If your space is small, the activity will work best when the children dance in their home spots. If the space is large enough for the children to move around, allow them to dance freely in the shared space. Play the song again while the children continue to respond to the music and their drawings.

Movement prompts in the song are:

• riding in the grocery cart

• pretending the cart is a rocket ship

• getting ready for a space trip

- counting down from ten to blastoff

- flying through outer space

- traveling through the stars

- looking at the planets

- landing on the moon

- heading for home

- going through the checkout line

Call out any or all of these prompts to spur more ideas while the children are dancing. Finish the activity by asking the children to imagine they are landing back on Earth, ending up in their home spots. To follow up on this imaginary adventure, the children may want to add more images to their drawings. They will have ideas from the movement and from the other children.

Modifications

A child can hold up pictures of the different parts of the activity, such as photos of a grocery store, rocket ships, and outer space, and he can lead the countdown by calling out the numbers. He can also sing along with the song.

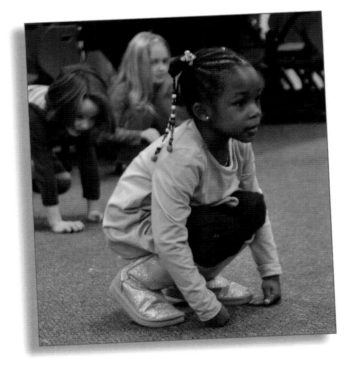

76

Dancing Statues

This activity incorporates a lively movement game with the learning of important national landmarks. Add your local favorites to the list too! The kinesthetic learning happens as the children attempt to make the shapes of the landmarks with their bodies.

Explores social studies!

What You Need

☼ a small space (the movement at the end of the activity can be done in place in a home spot or moving throughout the shared space)

☼ "Higgeldy Dance" instrumental (disc 2, track 25)

☼ pictures of the Statue of Liberty, Washington Monument, Lincoln Memorial, St. Louis Gateway Arch, and local landmarks

What You Do

To begin, show the children pictures of the landmarks and help them recognize and name them. Once they can, ask the children to spread out and find a home spot. Say to them:

Now we're going to dance about these statues and landmarks! While the music plays (play "Higgeldy Dance" instrumental), **you may dance freely. I'll stop the music while it's playing. When I do, I'll call out one of the statues: the Statue of Liberty, the Washington Monument, the Lincoln Memorial, the St. Louis Arch, or one of our local landmarks. You try to make the shape of the statue or landmark with your body, and hold that shape until the music begins again.**

Now we'll play this game a different way. I'd like everyone to return to their home spots. Now, staying in your spot, listen while I call out the names of the statues one by one. You make the shapes as soon as I say them.

Call out the names of the statues one by one, in random order, and ask the children to make the shapes in succession. Then ask the children to try it faster. Repeat, using a faster tempo each time.

We'll finish our game now. Take the shape of your favorite statue, and try to hold that shape as long as you can while you melt to the floor.

Modifications

A child can hold up the pictures of the statues and landmarks for you while the other children are becoming familiar with them. During the dance-and-freeze portion of the lesson, instead of calling out the statue cues yourself, allow the child to call them out or to hold the different pictures up as cues for the others as they make the shape of the corresponding statue or landmark.

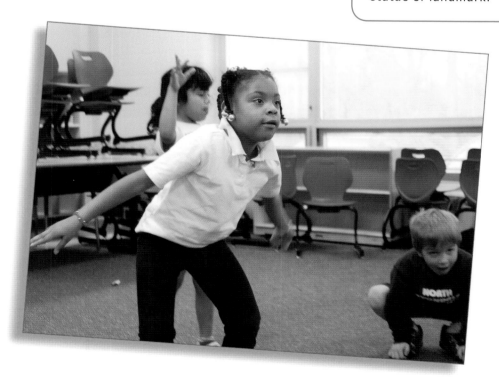

77

Let's Take a Bus Ride!

"Let's Take a Bus Ride!" is a good activity for familiarizing children with their immediate surroundings—they can travel on a bus anywhere their imaginations take them!

Explores social studies!

What You Need

☼ a large space

☼ "Savannah" instrumental (disc 2, track 35)

☼ a stop sign

What You Do

Place the children in home spots around the periphery of the room to begin the activity. Play "Savannah" instrumental quietly in the background. Say to the children:

Today we're going to take an imaginary bus ride around our town. I'll be the driver, and you'll be the riders. I'm going to pick you up one by one.

When I reach your bus stop, I'll stop and you'll climb on the bus. Once I've picked everyone up, we'll go around our town and I'll give you a tour.

A loosely gathered group of children begins following you as you stop for each child, and then continue all together.

Look, there's our library. Here's the park and the playground. Where else should we go on our tour?

We've seen so many places on our bus ride! I'll drop you off one by one back at your bus stop (the home spots). **Now we'll dance about all the sights we saw while taking our bus ride. Watch me for signals while you move.**

Hold up the stop sign and say to the children:

Does anyone know what this sign means? That's right, it means you must stop right away. When I hold the stop sign up, you must freeze! When I lower it, you may dance again. I'm going to put on some music, and when you hear it, you can dance freely.

Play "Savannah" instrumental again, louder. Hold and then lower the sign several times during the music. When the song comes to an end, hold the stop sign up one last time to signal the end of the dance.

Modifications

A child who uses a wheelchair can be a part of the bus ride. Assign another child or an aide to assist him in getting on and off the bus and to push him during the ride. During the free dance, a child can be assigned the job of "traffic director" and can hold the stop sign for the stop/go cues.

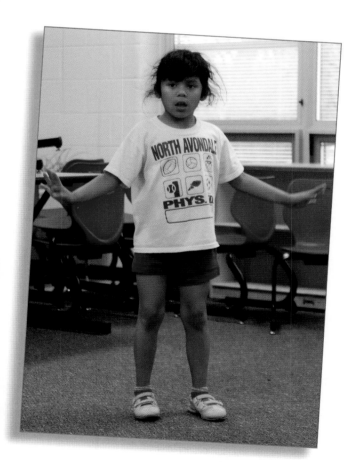

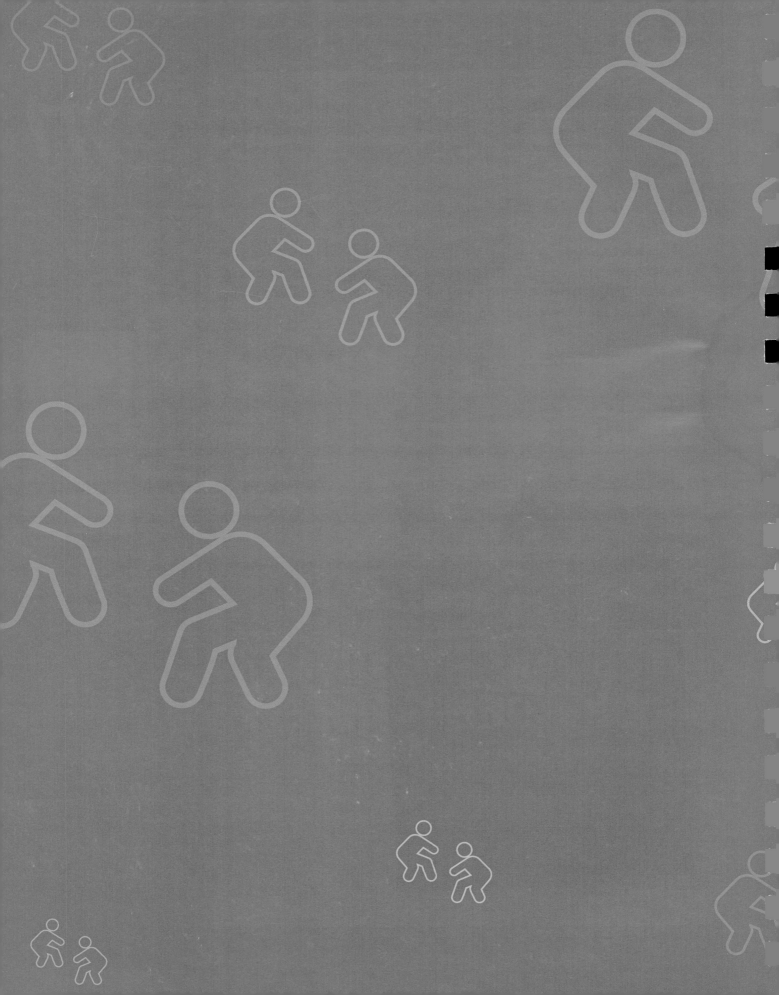

LOCOMOTION—LARGE-MOTOR SKILL ACTIVITIES

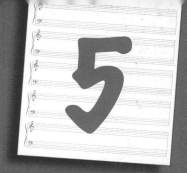

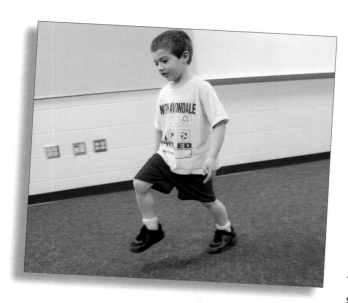

THE ACTIVITIES in "Locomotion—Large-Motor Skill Activities" are built around basic, age-appropriate locomotor (large-motor) skills—movements in which the feet take you from one place to another. The repetition and variations within the activities will help children acquire age-appropriate large-motor skills as well as reinforce and enhance the performance of the skills. All locomotor skills can be modified in many ways, using the elements of dance—body, time, space, and energy, as described in the introduction—to create fun tasks and games.

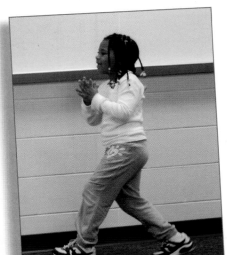

The activities in "Locomotion" are designed to be used in an open, unobstructed space, such as a gym or muscle room, or on a level outside space, such as a playground or lawn. You'll see that a few of the activities are designed specifically for older children, ages five and up. Regardless of age, it is important to note that not all children master skills at the same time. These activities allow children to try, practice, and eventually become proficient at the different skills.

The activities are organized into the following topics:

- **Walks and walk variations (activities 78 through 81)**

A walk is the most basic locomotor skill, consisting of a relaxed, regular stride, as alternating feet support the weight with each step. It is the foundation for other locomotor skills.

A march is a modified walk, performed with a different energy, rhythm, and stride, often with a high lift of the knee on the nonweight-bearing leg.

A lunge is a walk with a very large stride, usually with the supporting leg bent, and the nonweight-bearing leg relatively straight as it trails behind.

Tiptoe walks are walking steps using the metatarsals and toes of the supporting leg as the platform for the step, instead of using the whole foot, as in the basic walk.

- **Runs, prances, gallops, and slides (activities 82 and 83)**

A run is a modified walk (an even stride, alternating the weight-bearing leg with each step) performed at a faster pace, with more energy, and with both feet off the ground during the height of each stride.

A prance is a modified run, with both feet off the ground during the stride. The body is held straight and tall, and the bent knees are lifted in front of the body. The prance is very similar to the march step, with elevation off the ground during the weight change.

A gallop is a run with an uneven rhythm, consisting of one strong step and one lighter, less-accented step. The same foot leads throughout the gallop.

A slide is a sideways gallop, performed with the side of the body leading. Many steps in ballet are based on the slide. In ballet terminology, the slide is called a "chassé" (sha-*say*), or chasing step, as one leg leads and the other follows.

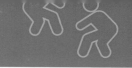
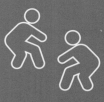

- **Jumps and hops (activities 84 through 86)**

All jumps and hops have a takeoff, an elevation, and a landing. A jump takes off and lands on two feet, and a hop takes off and lands on the same foot.

- **Skips and leaps—for children ages 5 and up (activities 87 and 88)**

A skip is a blended step, combining a walk step with a hop. The step-hop combination is performed on the same foot, and then alternates sides to create the lilting skip rhythm.

A leap is a modified run. During the transfer of weight from one leg to another, the body is high in the air, the take-off leg is stretched out behind the body, and the landing leg is stretched out in front of the body.

- **Free-movement explorations (activities 89 through 94)**

These activities provide additional opportunities for the children to practice large-motor skills doing fun, creative movement in a large space. The development of their motor skills will be reinforced as the children respond to the imaginative movement prompts.

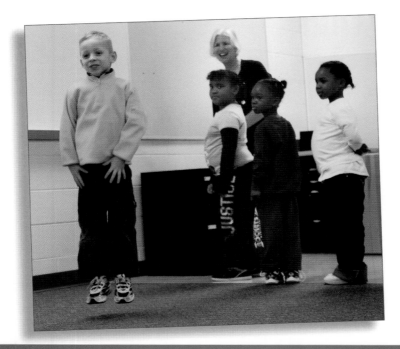

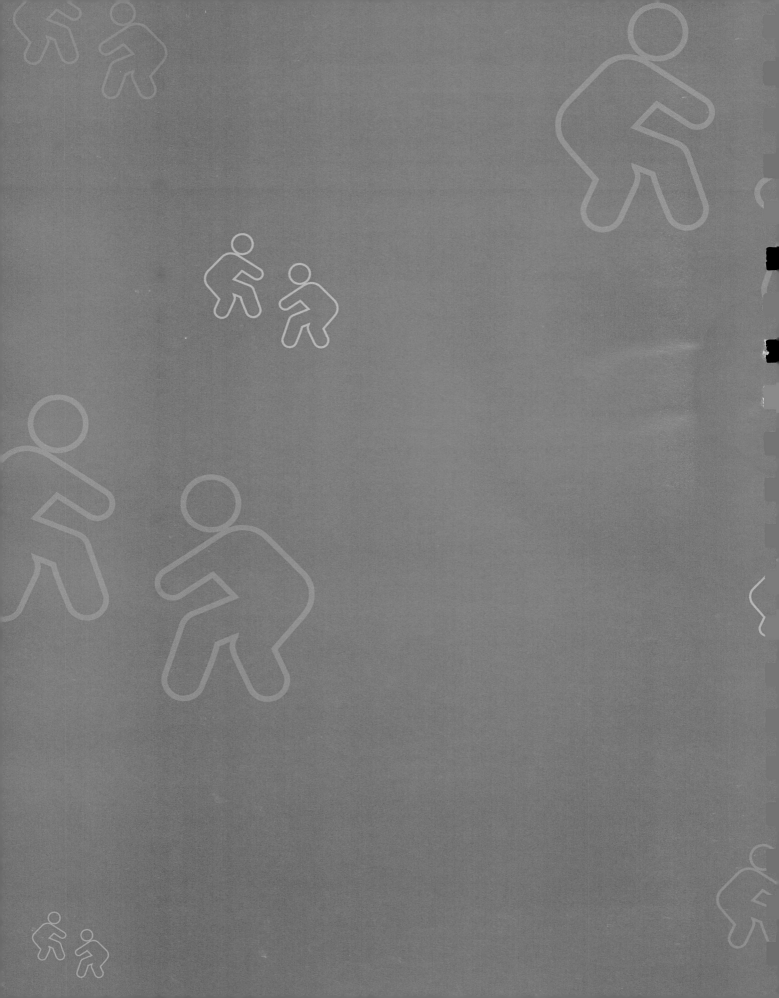

Baby Steps

"Baby Steps" is a playful activity designed for practicing the walk and for trying simple variations on the walking step. The children will begin with crawling, then standing, and working up to walking in different ways. They will enjoy thinking about when they were babies, and how many movements they can do now that they are bigger.

What You Need

☼ a large space, indoors

What You Do

Assign children home spots spread throughout the space. Say to the children:

Do you remember being a baby? Do you remember when you couldn't walk? What did you do? You crawled! Can you crawl like a baby? Try to crawl backward! Can you try to stand up?

Now imagine you can't walk very well. You take little baby steps, and you are pretty wobbly. Balance yourself by putting your hands out to the sides. Fall down on your seat and catch yourself with your hands. Now try to stand up again, and practice walking.

You are walking so well, just like you do every day, now that you are bigger! Walk all around the room. Swing your arms while you walk. Try giant steps now! Large steps with a bent front knee, which is what children usually do when they take giant steps, are called "lunges."

Let's go to one side of the room and line up side by side. Can you get all the way across the room in ten giant steps? Let's turn around and come back across the room using only baby steps.

78

Now, as we go across again, begin by walking with the regular steps we use when we walk to school or walk with a friend. Then I will say "giant steps" or "baby steps" or "regular steps," and you will walk in these different ways.

As long as the children are enjoying this activity, continue the back-and-forth movement across the floor, calling out different combinations of baby steps, giant steps, and normal walking steps.

Modifications

If a child is unable to participate in large-motor skill practice, then try including her in some of these ways. Bring pictures of a baby crawling, a baby pulling herself up to standing, and a child walking, and ask the child to hold the pictures up during the first part of the lesson, when the other children are crawling, standing up, and walking. You can also ask her to call out the different steps (baby steps, giant steps, or regular steps) in the latter part of the activity.

A child who uses a wheelchair can participate in the second part of the activity. For baby steps, she can go (or someone can push her) slowly; for regular steps, she can go at a normal pace; and for giant steps, she can go faster, equivalent to the pace of the children taking large steps.

Now let's finish our activity. Look at your home spot, and when I say "go," walk back to it taking giant steps. Are we all in our home spots? To finish our walking practice, let's all fall gently down on our seats, making sure to catch ourselves with our hands.

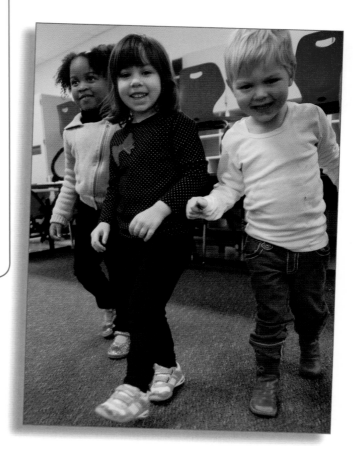

Cats and Lions on the Prowl

During "Cats and Lions on the Prowl," children will try several variations on walking: marching, tiptoe walking, and walking softly. The image of a cat helps them understand how to move quietly. At the end of the lesson, the children will practice pouncing like a cat and prowling like a lion.

What You Need

☼ a large space, indoors (the movement can be done outside if on a soft surface, such as grass)

☼ "Lion Prowl" instrumental (disc 2, track 28)

What You Do

Line the children up, side by side, with plenty of room between them, along one side of the space. They should be facing the space so that they can all go across at the same time. Say to them:

Let's practice moving like cats. We'll move from one side of the space to the other, and then back again, several times. Cats can be very quiet. They can move without making a sound. Can you walk softly like a cat all the way to the other side? Now let's turn around and come back across, trying that same quiet walk a little faster. Be sure to keep plenty of room between one another.

Now can you march softly? We will go across the space again, marching softly.

Now let's try walking high—go up on your tiptoes! Can you tiptoe all the way across, very quietly?

Repeat these motor skills—walking softly, marching softly, and tiptoeing—but a little faster. The children should finish on one side of the space in a line, with plenty of room between them, to be ready for the next part of the activity. Say to them:

Cats love to pounce, like when they're playing with a toy. When I call your name one by one, run about halfway to the other side and then pounce on your imaginary kitty toy!

Assign the children spots that are spread throughout the space for this second part of the activity. Say to them:

I am going to give you each a home spot for the next part of the activity. Tiptoe quietly as a cat to your new spot.

Cats and lions move in much the same way, don't they? They are in the same animal family. I'll put on some music, and you can practice moving like a cat. Try moving like a big lion, too, while you dance throughout the space. Play "Lion Prowl" instrumental.

How would a lion prowl as he sneaks through the tall grass? We will walk, march, tiptoe, and move like cats and lions now, but we won't pounce during the dance.

Modifications

Include a child in this activity by expanding the discussion about cats and lions. Bring pictures of each, and allow him to hold the pictures of the cat and lion while you discuss how a cat, and then a lion, moves.

Continue this free dance activity with the music, as long as the children are engaged. Finish the activity by saying:

We will do one more pounce to end this activity. Tiptoe back to your home spot. Do one big pounce onto your spot! Now sit down, and roll onto your side to rest like a big, sleepy lion.

Fun with Marching

"Fun with Marching" thoroughly explores the locomotor skill of marching, from feeling the beat, to transferring it into the body while marching, to refining the style of the step. A good follow-up to this is Activity 81: More Fun with Marching.

What You Need

- ☼ a large space, indoors or outside

- ☼ "Marching Band" instrumental (disc 2, track 30)

- ☼ a small drum or a tambourine (optional)

What You Do

Say to the children:

Let's all line up at one end of the space, side by side, with plenty of room between us. Listen to the steady beat as I tap on the drum. Can you clap the beat with me? Now we will feel the beat with our feet! Let's march across the floor together. Try to take one step each time I beat the drum. Let's turn around so we can cross back to the other side, still practicing taking one step for each drumbeat.

Now let's go across again, and I would like you to try lifting your knees high and landing lightly on the floor each time you step. Turn around and try the same thing as you go back to the other side. You are marching! This time when we go across and turn around and come back, swing your arms in a lively way when you march.

Now we will do something different with our arms. Can you clap on the beat as you march across and back? Now let's try marching for eight counts in a straight line, and then for eight counts in a small

80

circle around yourself. Now continue that—eight counts straight, eight counts in a small circle—all the way across the floor.

This time, march for four counts, and freeze for four counts, all the way across the floor. Can you balance on one leg during the freeze? Hold your arms out to the side during the freeze to help you balance.

Now we will try marching in slow motion to the other side. Turn around, and march back as fast as we can!

What was your favorite way of marching, of all of the different things we tried so far? Go across the floor with the march that you liked best.

I will put on some fun marching music (play "Marching Band" instrumental), and you can move around throughout the space trying all the marches one more time. When the music stops, freeze on one leg, and see if you can hold it while I count to ten!

Modifications

Ask a child to help you keep the beat of the steps. She can clap her hands, or hold the drum or tambourine, and will learn the skill of keeping a tempo and beat. She can also count to ten at the end of the lesson while the other children are holding their final positions.

More Fun with Marching

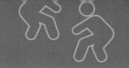

"More Fun with Marching" explores the energy of marching, and how it can be varied to change the movement quality of the march. Modifying the energy or force of a movement can result in imaginative and fun variations. This is a good follow-up to Activity 80: Fun with Marching.

What You Need

☼ a large space, indoors or outside

☼ "Higgeldy Dance" instrumental (disc 2, track 25)

☼ a small drum or a tambourine (optional)

What You Do

Say to the children:

Let's line up side by side at one end of the space, with plenty of room between one another. We'll go across the floor all together, turn around, and come back, marching to the beat. Listen to the beat for a few counts. If you have a drum or tambourine, use it to keep a steady beat. Or you can clap your hands.

Now I'll continue the beat, and we will count to ten together, and then we will start marching. Let's march across the floor, and turn around and come back, marching to the beat.

We are going to try some different ways of marching. I will call out an idea, and you try marching that way. Let's start by imagining that we just had a big rainstorm. We are going to stomp through the mud puddles! Stomping is like a very strong way of marching. Here we go!

Remember to step on the beat! Now let's turn around and stomp some more, all the way back to where we started.

This time we will march in a very different way. Try marching without making any noise. Go across the floor and then come back. See if you can do it very quietly. I will tap the beat quietly.

Next we will try another kind of marching. We will imagine that it is a very hot day. The sun is shining on a hot driveway. Let's pretend to take off our shoes. March across the room as if your feet are hot and can hardly touch the floor, then turn around and do the same thing going back.

Let's take an imaginary trip to the swamp. Put on your big boots. The mud and quicksand are deep! Try marching through that, as your feet get stuck each time. I am not going to keep a beat for this one, because you will need to stop and pull your boots out of the mud!

What would it be like to march underwater? Let's pretend to jump into a big lake. The water comes up to your shoulders. Now, march at your own speed as you push your legs through the water.

Continue this activity, with the children responding to each of your prompts as they move across the space and back again with each variation. Keep the beat if the prompt results in a steady marching step, such as marching like a wooden soldier. It is not necessary to keep the beat for all the variations, such as marching on the moon. Some more ideas are:

- **March and try to touch your knees to the sky.**

- **March on a slippery sidewalk.**

- **March as if you are a wooden soldier or robot.**

- **Imagine you are a robot and someone has set your controls so you march super-slowly, then super-fast, then try mixing them up, taking a few slow steps, and then a few quick steps.**

- **Imagine you are in a big space suit and you are trying to march on the moon!**

We have tried so many different kinds of marching! Now I'll play some music and you can try any of these ways of marching once again as you move around the space. Play "Higgeldy Dance" instrumental.

Let's sit down and try to march while we are sitting! Now we'll finish our marching fun by lying down on our backs and marching upside down!

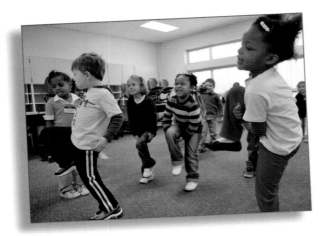

Modifications

A child who is unable to participate in the marching movements can help you keep the beat of the steps. He can clap his hands or hold the drum or tambourine, and will learn the skill of keeping a tempo and beat. You can also tell him each prompt that is coming up, and he can call them out at the beginning of the corresponding variation.

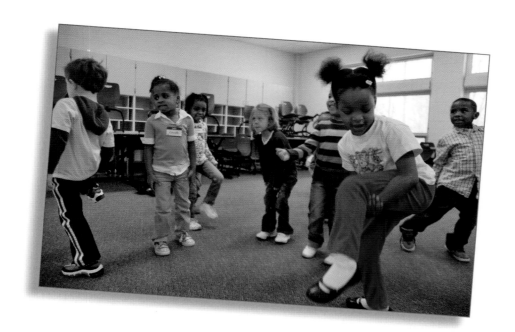

Walk, Trot, Prance, Gallop!

82

The progression of motor skills from walk, to trot, to prance, to gallop in this activity makes the gallop fun to learn and practice.

What You Need

☼ a large space, indoors or outside

☼ "Higgeldy Dance" instrumental (disc 2, track 25)

What You Do

To begin, spread the children evenly throughout the large space. Say to them:

Today we're going to think about how horses move. Let's all walk slowly, like a horse being led out of the barn. As you walk around the room, watch out for the other children as they move like big beautiful horses. It is a bright, sunny day on the ranch. What do you see as you look around?

Have you ever seen a horse trot? A trot is a very gentle, slow run. Let's trot like a horse!

Now let's try another way of trotting. Let's trot around the room some more, but this time, bring your knees up high in front of you with each step. You are prancing like a show horse!

Okay, horses, trot over to the side and line up, with plenty of space between each other. Let's think about the way horses run. Have you ever seen a horse gallop? Horses run smoothly and quickly when they gallop. Here is the rhythm of the gallop: one quick, soft clap, and one long, loud accented clap. Let's clap that rhythm together. Now let's gallop!

The children should take off on one foot and go up in the air on the long, loud clap, then land on the other foot on the quick clap. The same leg leads each step. Children should be encouraged to lead with whichever leg is comfortable for them. Once they are very familiar with the gallop step, you can suggest they try leading with one leg and then stop and try leading with the other.

Let's try it together, galloping across the room. And just like a horse slows down when someone pulls on the reins to guide him, we'll slow down and control our movement so we come to a gentle stop at the other side of the room. First we'll clap the gallop rhythm four times together, and then we'll step and take off on the loud clap and land on the other foot on the quiet clap. Let's gallop together across the room. Here we go! Now slow down as you imagine someone pulling on your reins!

Okay, horses, turn around and go back the same way. Let's do that a few more times. What do you see as you gallop across the field? Try clapping your hands along with the galloping rhythm as you go.

Here are more galloping movement prompts:

- **Can you gallop higher on the strong clapping beat?**

- **Can you take bigger galloping steps? Let's try to cross the space in ten gallops! Let's count together while we gallop. Now let's try to cross the floor in nine gallops! Let's try eight!**

Modifications

Children who have difficulty with this large-motor skill activity can participate by helping keep the beat with small percussion instruments while the other children are doing the various steps. They can also help you count while the others are doing specific numbers of gallops.

- **Let's imagine we are cowboys. What do cowboys do while they gallop on their horses? Do they swing a rope? Can you try that?**

- **What would it feel like to be the horse with a cowboy riding on your back?**

- **Can you gallop in a great big circle? Can you turn around and gallop the other way in a big circle?**

Spread out through the space, and now we will move freely to some music. I will play a song that has a galloping beat. Play "Higgeldy Dance" instrumental. **You may practice the walk, trot, prance, and gallop steps, and dance about all of the ideas we had about being cowboys and horses.**

Now let's bring our galloping fun to an end. Imagine you're a horse who's been galloping all day. Let's slow down to a prance, and then relax as you come to a slow trot. Now we will slow down to a nice, easy walk. Aren't you ready to go back to the barn to rest and eat some hay?

83

The Dancing Letter "H"

The slide, or "chassé" (sha-say), is a gallop performed with the side of the body leading the movement. Children usually catch on to slides very quickly, especially when they become familiar with the rhythm. Once they begin to master the step, many fun activities can follow, as in the variations suggested in the lesson. This is a good follow-up to Activity 39: Action Alphabet "H."

What You Need

☼ a large space, indoors or outside

☼ "It's Preschool" instrumental (disc 2, track 26)

☼ a small drum or a tambourine (optional)

What You Do

Divide the children into pairs. Space the pairs evenly across one side of the area. The children will face each other, standing so that when they begin the sideways slide, they will be moving across the floor face to face, traveling by leading with the side of the body facing the open space.

The slide is a gallop performed sideways, leading with the side of the body instead of the front. Its rhythm is the same as the rhythm for a gallop: one soft beat and one loud beat. If you have a drum or tambourine, beat the rhythm of the step. If you don't, clap your hands instead. The children will move in pairs, either one pair at a time or all of the pairs together spread out across the room. Ask a child to demonstrate the movement with you before everyone tries it, or try it with each child before pairing the children together. Say to them:

We're going to practice a fun movement today called the slide. Let's clap the rhythm of the slide movement. The rhythm is like a horse

galloping: one soft, quick clap, and one long, loud clap. Let's clap this rhythm together: soft-loud, soft-loud, soft-loud—and keep it going!

Now face your partner. Open your arms to the side and try to stay across from your partner as you slide all the way to the other side of the space. While I continue to clap the beat, I'd like you to move sideways together, sliding the beat in your feet: soft-loud, soft-loud. As you hear the soft beat, step and bend your knees. As you hear the loud beat, travel with the sideways slide step toward the other side, trying to touch your feet together in the air. Keep it going all the way across the room.

Now we'll try it with each pair holding hands, making a great big letter "H." Each of you makes one side of the "H," and together your hands make the line that joins the two long lines. As you go across the floor with your partner, look at each other and try to move together. Don't pull each other's hands, just hold them, and see if you can stay exactly together. Make sure you slow down before you reach the other side of the space.

Next let's try some variations. Imagine you are holding a great big ball as you slide across the floor facing your partner. The children should open their arms wide, forming a large imaginary circle between them. Now try a pumpkin, and then a great big snowball. What else would you and your partner like to hold while you slide together?

Smile at your partner the whole time you're sliding across the space together. This time make silly faces at one another while you slide. Hold your arms out to the side, as you did before.

Can you slide back to back with your partner? Don't touch your partner while you do this, but try to stay with him just as you did when you were facing each other, and hold your arms out to the side.

Let's make two rows of children facing each other. This will be our tunnel. Each pair will take a turn sliding down the middle of our tunnel. When you reach the end, become part of the tunnel again. Let's do it again, and when you are part of the tunnel, clap the soft-loud rhythm pattern of the slide step.

83

Let's do slides one by one across the floor now, with music! Line the children up across one side of the space, and call their names one by one. Do this several times, back and forth across the space. Play "It's Preschool" instrumental.

Do you remember how we began this activity? You were lined up on this side of the space facing your partner. Can you walk back to that spot? Now face your partner and do a big bow to each other!

Modifications

Children who have difficulty with this large-motor skill activity can still participate by helping keep the beat (with small percussion instruments) while the other children are doing the slides. They can participate in the tunnel activity, first by being part of the tunnel, and then by taking a turn going down the tunnel with any movement they choose.

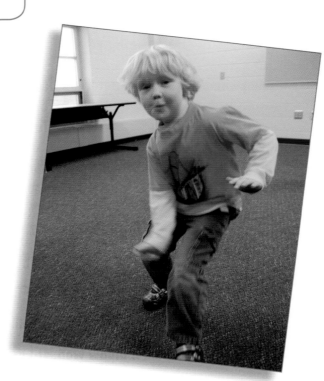

Bend and Balance, Jump and Hop

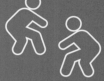

These exercises are designed to teach the correct technique for any movement that leaves the floor to go up in the air. The bending and stretching of the legs, holding the body correctly, and practicing balancing sets the stage for the children to jump with proper takeoffs and landings. Good follow-up activities to this lesson are Activity 85: Jumping Fun and Activity 86: Jumpin' Jiminy Jamboree. This is a good lead-in to Activity 88: Learning to Leap (for children ages five and up).

What You Need

☼ a small space

What You Do

Stand in a circle so all of the children can see each other and watch as you demonstrate the movements for them. After you have demonstrated the movements, ask the children to do them along with you.

Knee Bends and Tiptoe Balances

Stand with your feet parallel to each other and about hip-width apart. Bend your knees, maintaining contact between your heels and the floor, and then straighten your legs, coming back up from the knee bend and resuming a normal stance. Keep your back straight and upright throughout the knee bend. Do this slowly and prompt the children to do it along with you several times.

To help children balance while they do a knee bend, ask them to imagine they are hugging a great big beach ball, keeping their arms in a wide, slightly rounded position. (Holding their arms in a specific position allows children to concentrate on their bodies and legs and helps them balance.) Try several more knee bends with them as they hold their arms in this position.

Next, straighten your legs, rise up on the balls of your feet, and try to balance for one or two seconds. Remind the children that they are still holding a big beach ball in order to maintain the specific arm position, as they do this along with you.

Now do a knee bend and straighten up directly into a tiptoe balance, and then come back down to a knee bend without stopping in between. Do this a few times, and end by trying to balance on tiptoes.

Jumps and Hops

A bent-knee position is the most important part of a jump: it assures a good takeoff and a soft, safe landing. In addition to maintaining bent knees, children should not land flat-footed; toes should touch first, and then, in rapid succession, the balls of the feet and finally the heels.

Jump up and down while beginning and ending in the knee-bend position, and hold your arms wide and rounded in front. Ask the children to follow along with you, holding their arms in front: "Don't drop your beach ball!" Start out with small bouncy jumps, and then work up to higher, bigger jumps.

Next say to the children:

A hop is a kind of jump, but do you know what the difference is? A hop is a jump on one foot! Let's try our little bouncy jumps on one foot, and then on the other. Let's do four on each foot. Hold your imaginary beach ball to help you balance! Let's end our hopping by doing one big one, and try to balance on that foot when you land. Try the same thing on the other foot.

Let's finish with some big jumps. They are just the same as the little ones, always beginning and ending with bent knees, but we will use lots of energy and jump higher. Let's do six big jumps all together!

As children begin to master jumps and hops, they should try to hold their bodies straight and tall throughout the jump and hop, and the landing should be quiet. Children who are five years old and up should work toward the correct way to land from a jump or any airborne movement.

Here are some prompts you can use for both jumps and hops as you continue the activity:

- **Can you make a funny face each time you jump (or hop)?**

- **Can you make a shape with your arms while you jump (or hop)?**

- **Can you jump (or hop) four times and make four different shapes with your arms?**

- **What different shapes can you make with your whole body while you're in the air?**

- **Can you jump (or hop) backward?**

- **Can you balance on one foot when you land from your hop? Can you do the same thing on the other foot?**

- **Can you jump (or hop) and turn around?**

- **Can you land from your jumps and hops without making any noise?**

- **Can you lie on the floor and hop upside down?**

Modifications

A jump or hop is an up-and-down movement, and children can try it with other parts of the body. Encourage them to try the up-and-down movement with their head, eyelids, mouth, shoulders, elbows, wrists, hands, arms, legs, feet, and toes, moving one (or more than one) part at the same time. Prompt them to use any and all of these parts of the body they can, and to try to keep the beat as they do so.

85

Jumping Fun
• • • • • • • • •

It is important for children to learn to jump properly, so present Activity 84: Bend and Balance, Jump and Hop, before proceeding to this one. "Jumping Fun" continues the exploration of this motor skill, using examples of jumping in the animal kingdom and in common activities and games. More ideas using this motor skill can be found in Activity 86: Jumpin' Jiminy Jamboree.

What You Need

☼ a large space, indoors or outside

What You Do

Ask the children to stand in a circle. Instruct them to bend their knees and then stretch up onto their tiptoes eight to ten times, to warm up for jumps. Say to them:

Can you name some animals that can jump? Frogs, rabbits, kangaroos, grasshoppers, crickets, horses, kittens, and dolphins all can jump. Can you imagine how they jump? For instance, cats can jump very high, like when they jump up onto a tall counter or chair. How high can you jump? Give it a try! Can you jump three times in a row, as high as you can? Can you try it again? At the end of your last jump, make your favorite kitty shape and freeze.

Now ask the children to line up, side by side, on one side of the room, with plenty of space between them. Say to them:

Let's try moving across the floor together, jumping like some of the animals we mentioned.

Staying in your place in our long line, let's run until we are halfway across. When we reach that point, let's stop and do a big jump like a frog when I clap my hands. Then we'll walk to the other side.

Now let's turn around and do the same thing, except this time we'll imagine a rabbit instead of a frog. Run halfway across the space, jump like a rabbit when I clap my hands, and then walk to the other side.

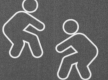

Continue this format until you have used all of the animal examples, and let the children contribute their own if they want to add some more. When you are finished, place the children in home spots spread evenly throughout the space. Allow each of the ideas in this next section to unfold so the children have the opportunity to explore each one. Say to the children:

People love to jump too! Let's think of some of the games and activities people do with jumps and hops—pogo stick, jump rope, hopscotch, jumping jacks, basketball, and dancing, to name a few. Let's try each of these ideas one by one. Can you jump on an imaginary pogo stick in your home spot? Can you jump six times? Now take an imaginary jump rope and think about turning it so you can jump over it. Hopscotch has jumps and hops in it. Let's try jump, hop, jump, hop, jump, freeze! Now let's try some jumping jacks. Can you do them while you are turning around?

Imagine you are holding a basketball, and jump high while you are trying to make a basketball shot. Now dance in your spot, and try dancing while you jump and hop. Do you want to try any other jumping ideas?

That was a lot of jumping, so let's do a quiet finish. Go down to the floor, sit in your home spot, and put your legs straight out in front of you. Bend your head and neck forward gently, just a little bit, and breathe while you relax your muscles. Slowly lift your neck and head back up so you are sitting tall. Let's repeat that easy breathing movement a few times to relax after all that jumping.

Modifications

A jump or hop is an up-and-down movement, and children can try it with other parts of the body. Encourage them to try the up-and-down movement with their head, eyelids, mouth, shoulders, elbows, wrists, hands, arms, legs, feet, and toes, moving one (or more than one) part at the same time. Prompt them to use any and all of these parts of the body they can, and to try to keep the beat as they do so.

86

Jumpin' Jiminy Jamboree

· · · · · · · · · · · · · ·

It is important for children to learn to jump properly, so present Activity 84: Bend and Balance, Jump and Hop, before proceeding to this one. More ideas for using this motor skill can be found in Activity 85: Jumping Fun.

What You Need

☼ a large space

☼ "Jumpin' Jiminy" (disc 1, track 8)

What You Do

Ask the children to sit in a circle, with plenty of room between each one. Instruct them to bend their knees and then stretch up onto their tiptoes eight to ten times, to warm up for jumps. Say to them:

Here's a fun song that has a great jumping beat. It also has lots of "J" sounds in it. See if you can hear them. Listen for the bouncy, jumping beat too. Play "Jumpin' Jiminy."

Now we will stand up in our places in the circle. I will play the music again. We will move to the words of the song. When the song tells us to jump, beginning with the words, "Jumpin' Jiminy Jamboree," you may jump and hop in your spot, and turn in place while you are jumping and hopping. When the music slows down, take a rest, breathe, and move slowly, listening to the words in the song and waiting for the jumping beat again. When the "Jumpin' Jiminy" words are repeated, do jumps and hops again along with the song. When you

hear the words, "Girls and boys from wide and far, our game is done, you were a star," slowly melt to the floor.

Now let's do our "Jumpin' Jiminy" dance one more time! This time, you will spread out in the space to begin, and you may move around the space while you jump, hop, turn, and dance to the song. At the end, we will jump back to our home spots and slowly melt to the floor, just like we did before.

Modifications

A jump or hop is an up-and-down movement, and children can try it with other parts of the body. Encourage them to try the up-and-down movement with their head, eyelids, mouth, shoulders, elbows, wrists, hands, arms, legs, feet, and toes, moving one (or more than one) part at the same time. Prompt them to use any and all of these parts of the body they can, and to try to keep the beat as they do so.

Encourage the children to sing along to the words of "Jumpin' Jiminy," once they have become familiar with the song.

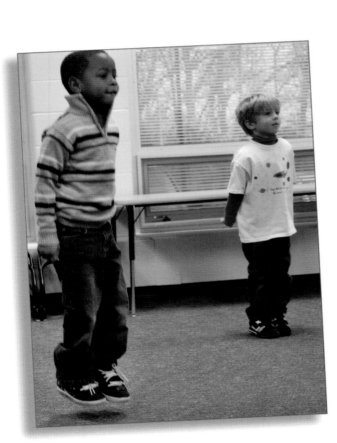

Step, Hop, Skip, Skip, Skip!

87

Children who are five years old can begin to learn the locomotor skill of skipping. Skipping steps are a combination of a forward walking step and a hop. This pattern then alternates on each leg and creates the easy, lilting rhythm of the skip. Children will acquire this skill at different rates, but because the rhythm for the skip is the same as the gallop rhythm, everyone can participate in the activities of this lesson, with some children skipping while others may be galloping. Repetition of the practice exercises, such as the clapping of the rhythm, and doing the skill slowly, will help the children to learn this locomotor skill.

What You Need

- ☼ a large space, indoors or outside

- ☼ "It's Preschool" instrumental (disc 2, track 26)

- ☼ a drum or a tambourine (optional)

What You Do

Line up the children, side by side, along one side of the space. Make sure there is plenty of room between them. Use the drum or tambourine, or clap your hands, to tap out the rhythm. The rhythm for a skip is one quick, soft clap and one long, loud accented clap. This rhythm pattern is continually repeated. Say to the children:

Let's learn to skip. Watch me do some slow skipping, and see if you can guess what movements make up a skip. Yes, first a step, and then, on the same foot, a hop. After that, I do the same thing on the other foot. Let's try it all together now, slowly: step, hop, step, hop, step, hop—all the way across the floor.

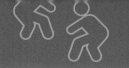

Now let's stand still for a minute and clap the rhythm of a skip. We will clap one quick, soft clap, and one long, loud accented clap. As we clap, let's say out loud: "Step hop, step hop, step hop, step hop, and skip, and skip, and skip, and skip." I will say those rhythm words again a few more times, and you try to clap and say them with me.

Now turn around and let's go back across the floor. I'll say the rhythmic words, and you try to skip while listening to the rhythm. Here we go! Step hop, step hop, step hop, step hop, and skip, and skip, and skip, and skip!

Repeat this several times, with the children skipping back and forth across the floor, accompanied by your rhythmic words and clapping.

Now we'll try it with the music. First let's listen to "It's Preschool" instrumental to hear the beat, and then let's skip across the floor with the music.

Some children will learn to skip right away, and others will take much longer to catch on, possibly doing the gallop step instead of the skip. Many will be able to perform the alternating step, hop, step, hop, but will not be able to integrate them into a lilting, rhythmic skip. With practice, as well as with hearing the skipping rhythm in your voice, the drumbeat, and the music, most children who are five years or older will eventually master this motor skill.

Try these movement prompts to add variety and challenge to the practice of skipping:

- **Can you skip and swing your arms?**

- **How high can you skip?**

- **Can you skip in a circle?**

- **Can you bring your knees up high?**

- **Can you clap the rhythm while you skip?**

- **Let's imagine it's a beautiful summer day, and we're skipping through a meadow of wildflowers!**

Modifications

Children who have difficulty with this large-motor skill activity can still participate by helping keep the beat with small percussion instruments while the other children are learning and practicing the skip. Another idea to include children is to let them call out the prompts for the skipping practice, such as "How high can you skip?" and "Can you skip in a circle?"

88 Learning to Leap

Children who are five years old can begin to learn the locomotor skill of leaping. A leap is actually one high, wide running step, which takes off from one leg, goes up into the air, and lands on the other leg, which bends on contact with the floor to soften the landing. When learning leaps, it is helpful for the children to imagine leaping over something, such as a rainbow, a river, or a fence. The leap is a lively motor skill children love to practice, so many ideas for developing and refining the skill are offered in this lesson. It is important for children to learn to warm up and jump properly, so present Activity 84: Bend and Balance, Jump and Hop before this one.

What You Need

☼ a large space, indoors or outside

☼ "Celebrate" instrumental (disc 1, track 18)

☼ a drum or a tambourine; masking tape or string (optional); a photo of a runner or dancer leaping (optional)

What You Do

Prepare the space by placing a long strip of masking tape or string across the center of the floor, if the space can accommodate this arrangement. Line up the children, side by side, along one side of the space. Make sure there is plenty of room between them. Instruct the children to bend their knees and then stretch up onto their tiptoes several times, and then run in place, to warm up for runs and leaps. Say to the children:

Today we are going to learn to leap. Have you ever seen a horse leap over a fence? She jumps very high and stretches out her legs so that

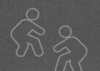

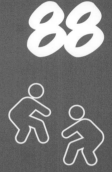

she looks like she is flying! People can leap too. Look at this picture of a dancer leaping. His legs are reaching long and straight, and look how high he is off the ground!

Here is the rhythm we will use for leaps. Clap along with me: 1, 2, 3, 4, 5, 6, 7, 8. (Accent beats 7 and 8.)

Repeat this several times, and then change the numbers to words: "run, run, run, run, run, run, HIGH LEAP!" Do this, too, several times and clap along with your words. Continue by saying to the children:

Do you see the tape along the center of the floor? Let's imagine the tape is a fence, and we are going to leap over that fence. Remember our rhythm? You will take running steps when I say "run, run, run, run, run, run," and then everybody will take a great big leap over the tape when I say "HIGH LEAP!" After you leap and land, slow down your run and put on your brakes to stop as you get to the other side.

Here we go: run, run, run, run, run, run, HIGH LEAP! Slow down and line up on the other side to try it again. Repeat a few more times.

An image that helps children leap is the idea of taking a photograph. Tell them you will take an imaginary photograph of them when they are in the air at the highest point of their leap. This will help the children begin to refine the form of the leap, which should have the front leg reaching forward in the air, and the back leg reaching back. The landing should be quiet and light, on the front leg first, with a soft, easy knee bend.

Let's keep leaping! Instead of my tambourine (or drum or hand clap), we'll use the beat of the music to help us know when to leap. Let's listen to the music first. While we listen, we'll count just like we did before: run, run, run, run, run, run, HIGH LEAP!

Play "Celebrate" instrumental, and have the children move across the space all together, leaping on counts seven and eight of the music. Repeat this a few times. Then say:

88

Next let's go across the floor with the music, one at a time. Everyone who is watching will say "run, run, run, run, run, run, HIGH LEAP!" for the person who is practicing her leaps. Repeat for each child.

Children will develop the skill of leaping at different rates, with some wanting to take off and/or land on two feet. The image of the photograph taken at the height of their leaps, the tape or the imaginary object they are leaping over, the picture of the dancer or runner, and the repetition of the practice of leaps will help children develop this skill. It is not necessary to concentrate on what the arms do while the children are first learning to leap; this is a detail that can be added later. Use the many ideas below to practice and vary the leaps, trying different ideas on different days, to help children to become proficient at this skill.

- **Can you leap higher? The fence is taller now! Leap over the rainbow!**

- **Can you leap farther? The river is even wider! The pile of leaves is getting bigger!**

- **What else can you leap over?**

- **Imagine you are holding a big ball in front of you. While you are running, throw it into the air at the top of your leap, and catch it when you land!** This prompt helps the children with body awareness and control throughout the whole exercise.

Modifications

Children who have difficulty with this large-motor skill activity can still participate in the lesson by helping tap the beat with small percussion instruments while the other children are learning and practicing leaps. Bring pictures of horses and other animals leaping, and pictures of objects to leap over, such as rainbows, fences, rivers, and leaf piles. Allow the children to hold up the pictures as the others are leaping, and to call out the prompts: "Imagine you are a tiger leaping over a river," or "Can you leap over this great big pile of leaves?"

Opposites

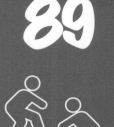
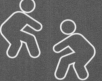

Movement opposites like "stomp" and "sneak," set into rhyme, provide the backdrop for this lively activity. New words like "scurry," "centipede," and "lumber" are introduced. The children can learn about opposites, and the meaning of the new words, while trying out the playful movements. Two more activities that addresses the theme of opposites are Activity 19: Big Green Alligator and Activity 22: Fast and Slow, High and Low.

What You Need

☼ a small space, indoors or outside (the free dance at the end of the activity can be done moving throughout the shared space)

What You Do

Begin with the children seated in a circle or in a home spot throughout the room. Read "Opposites" to them.

Opposites

March straight like a soldier
Hup, two, three!
Then slouch like a scarecrow
Loose as can be.

Soar high like an eagle
Wind under wing.
Crawl low like a centipede
a hundred-legged thing.

Scurry like a busy bee
Buzzing to the hive.
Lumber like a turtle
To the pond and dive.

Wide is the great big whale
Swim, roll, glide,
Narrow is the skinny eel
Slither, slip, slide.

Stomp loudly like an elephant
With big heavy feet.
Sneak like a tiger
Feel your heart beat.

Once you have read the poem through, read each stanza one by one, pointing out the opposites, and talk about any unfamiliar words or phrases. Then say to the children:

Let's stand up and dance the poem. I will read it slowly, and you will move to the words.

March straight like a soldier
Hup, two, three!

- standing tall, march in place; repeat, marching in a small circle, salute, and stop

Then slouch like a scarecrow
Loose as can be

- flop the upper body over and move around the spot with a slouchy, floppy quality

Soar high like an eagle
Wind under wing.

- make a small circle around the spot, using arms as wings; then do it in the other direction

Crawl low like a centipede
a hundred-legged thing

- go onto all fours and crawl around the spot, imagining you have lots of legs

Scurry like a busy bee
Buzzing to the hive.

- move like a bumblebee flying in a quick, zigzag pattern; make a buzzing sound

Lumber like a turtle
To the pond and dive.

- walk slowly, heavily like a turtle with his big shell on his back; at the home spot, take one high jump and land in an imaginary pond

Wide is the great big whale
Swim, roll, glide.

- pretend to be a whale, swimming, rolling, jumping, and flipping its tail

Narrow is the skinny eel
Slither, slip, slide.

- swim like an eel, turning, darting quickly, slipping through narrow spaces

Stomp loudly like an elephant
With big heavy feet

- imagine being big and heavy like an elephant; stomp around the home spot

Sneak like a tiger
Feel your heart beat.

- tiptoe quietly around the home spot; put hand on chest to feel heartbeat

Modifications

Invite the child to help you call out the words of the poem while the others move. Prompt her quietly with the words line by line, then have her repeat them aloud to the group along with you. Bring pictures of the various images in the poem—a soldier, a scarecrow, an eagle—for the child to hold up during the corresponding parts of the poem.

Repeat the activity if the children are still engaged. This time allow the children to leave their home spots and dance freely throughout the shared space as they respond to the prompts. Encourage them to try new movement ideas for each one. Finish by asking the children to sit quietly in their home spots, breathing and listening to the beat of their hearts.

89

90

Who Am I?

"Who Am I?" is a very open-ended activity, using movements generated by the children's own ideas and preferences. You can guide them or let their imaginations run freely as the activity develops.

What You Need

☼ a large space

☼ "Happy Face" (disc 1, track 6), "Kweezletown" instrumental, "Monster Spray" instrumental, or "Zoo Babies" instrumental (disc 2, tracks 27, 31, or 42)

What You Do

Begin the activity with the children in home spots spread throughout the space. Say to them:

Let's imagine we can transform into different people, characters, animals, or superheroes. Who or what would you like to be? Let's share our ideas with one another.

As the children present their ideas one by one, prompt them to imagine the different characteristics—what would they look like, what would they wear, and how would they move? For example, for a child who selects Raggedy Andy, you can say:

- **What clothes does Raggedy Andy wear?**

- **Is his face happy or sad?**

- **What color is his hair?**

- **If a rag doll came to life, how would it dance? It would be loose and floppy, wouldn't it?**

Play one of the musical selections, and ask all of the children to dance their character. They can move freely throughout the space, and when they are finished, ask them to return to their home spots.

Next ask another child for an idea and help him develop it with prompts similar to the ones suggested above. Play one of the musical selections and allow all of the children to dance about the idea. Continue this until each child has contributed an idea. Then proceed to the next part of the lesson. Say to the children:

We will have one more chance to dance about all of the ideas we had! I will put on some music (play one of the selections), **and you can dance about your own idea, about any of the ideas of the other children, and about any new ideas you might have about people, animals, characters, or superheroes. Move freely throughout the space. When the music ends, return to your home spot and freeze in the shape of your favorite character!**

Continue the activity as long as it holds the children's interest. If you decide to offer this activity often, consider narrowing the categories. For instance, you can focus in on animals one day and characters or superheroes another day, to go along with a theme, story, or book you're studying.

Modifications

An open-ended activity such as this one allows children who have physical limitations to use their imaginations to become anything they wish. A child who is blind or visually impaired could be Superman with X-ray vision, and she can dance about that idea within a small space laid out with safe boundaries, such as a textured mat that delineates the dancing area. A child who cannot walk can imagine he is flying on a magic carpet, doing whatever movements he can with his body while his mind takes him up into the sky. Encourage all children to participate in this activity, and prompt them with ideas: "Imagine you are Spiderman and can swing from tall buildings!" or "What if you could be a character from your favorite book?"

91

Go and Stop

• • • • • • • • • • •

The short poem "Go and Stop" will inspire a fun game of dance and freeze. The children's own ideas for how to "go" will create imaginative movement combinations!

What You Need

☼ a large space, indoors or outside

☼ "Dance S'More" instrumental (disc 1, track 20)

What You Do

The children begin seated in home spots spread throughout the space. Read the poem to the children:

Go and Stop

How many ways can we say go?
Slide, jog, prance, trot—faster please!
How many ways can we say stop?
Halt, pause, finish, stand still, and freeze!

Say to the children:

What words were used for "go" in the poem? Can you think of other ways that you can "go"? Good examples are "walk," "hop," "crawl," "gallop." **What words in the poem were used for "stop"? Yes! All of those words mean the same thing! Now we will play a game about "go" and "stop."**

Let's review all of the words we discovered that are ways to "go." I will play the music (play "Dance S'More" instrumental), **and you can do any of the "go" movements, moving freely throughout the shared space. When I stop the music, you freeze! See if you can stand still, and try not to move a muscle!**

Play the music again if the children are still engaged in the activity. Finish with them prancing back to their home spots. Ask them to freeze when they arrive at their spots, holding for ten counts as you count aloud together.

Modifications

Invite the child to help you call out the words of the poem. Quietly prompt him with the words to each line, and then invite him to call them out to the group with you. Ask the child who cannot participate in the movement to start and stop the music while the other children dance.

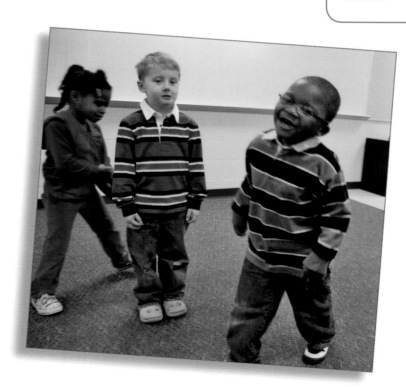

Rock Stars

• • • • • • • • • •

"Rock Stars" is a simple game of move and freeze. The children will use their imaginations as they dance about, playing the guitar, drums, and keyboard, and singing with a microphone.

What You Need

☼ a small space (the free dance at the end of the activity can be done moving throughout the shared space)

☼ "Celebrate" instrumental (disc 1, track 18)

What You Do

Ask everyone to find home spots spread throughout the space. Say to the children:

This game is about imagining you're in a rock band! There are five movement ideas for the dancing part of the activity:

- **playing imaginary drums**

- **playing air guitar**

- **playing keyboard**

- **holding a microphone and pretending to sing**

- **clapping your hands while you dance**

I will play some music and call out one of the five movements, such as "Play air guitar!" and you will do that movement in your home spot to the music. When I stop the music, freeze in your last shape! I'll then call out one of the other five movements, such as "Hold a microphone and pretend to sing!" and when I start the music again, you can dance about that idea.

Play "Celebrate" instrumental. Call out the five movement prompts in random order, using all of them at least once during the music, while the children respond. Repeat this part of the activity if the children are still engaged. To continue the activity, ask the children to stand in their home spots. Tell them that when the music starts, they can dance throughout the space. Say to them:

Now I will play the music all the way through one more time and you can dance freely around the room. Use all of the rock star movements we've practiced so far—and anything else that reminds you of being in a rock band!

Modifications

If children are unable to do the large movements in this activity, let them try all of the activities sitting or lying down rather than standing. Another idea is to give them a tambourine or small drum to play along with the music.

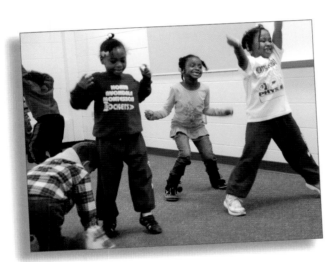

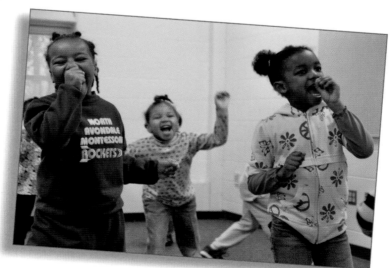

Straight, Flop

• • • • • • • • • • •

"Straight, Flop" is a lively activity using a poem as the prompt. Children learn to repeat the poem first, and then they learn the movements. Once they have mastered the words and movements, they can perform them together. "Straight, Flop" can be used for a quick movement break between other activities. The last section adds the element of large-motor skills practice to the activity.

What You Need

☼ a small space, indoors or outside (the variation at the end of the activity can be done moving throughout the shared space)

☼ a tambourine or a small drum (optional)

What You Do

The children can stand in a circle or home spots scattered throughout the room. Begin by reciting the poem to the children.

Straight, Flop

A bunny on the road
Went hop, hop, hop.
His ears were straight
And then they went flop!
Straight, flop, straight, flop,
Turn, jump, drop!

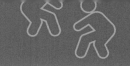

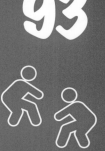

Then teach the movements that accompany the words:

A bunny on the road

- reach your arms up high

Went hop, hop, hop.

- hold your arms up, and hop three times in your spot

His ears were straight

- freeze, hold your body straight and arms up

And then they went flop!

- body and arms flop over; bend from the waist

Straight, flop, straight, flop,

- body straight, bend to flop position, straight, bend to flop position

Turn, jump, drop!

- turn around quickly, jump into the air, and land in a low crouch

Repeat several times in a row. To finish, add "Flop!" to the last verse. The children can end in a sitting position or lying on the floor.

For a variation, integrate locomotor movements to create a lively game out of "Straight, Flop." Use a tambourine or small drum to keep the beat during the transitions, or clap your hands.

Start the children in home spots with plenty of room between them. Along with the children, say the poem and do the movements again. After "drop" in the last line, call out and clap or tap (on the tambourine or drum) an eight-count transition. With their arms down by their sides, the children should walk, taking a step on each beat of the rhythm you are clapping or tapping. Invite them to count aloud with you while they walk. Then recite the poem and perform the movements all together once more. Repeat this pattern as long as the children are engaged.

93

To end the activity, ask the children to return to their home spots during the last eight-count transition. Repeat the poem one last time, and after "drop," say "Flop!" to prompt the children to finish in a seated position.

To add a challenge to the game, vary the transition movement. Ask the children to jump, hop, take giant steps, march, prance, or tiptoe instead of walk. Call out the new locomotor movement before each transition.

Modifications

Invite the child to help you call out the words of the poem while the others are moving. Quietly prompt her with the words before you say each line, and then have her repeat them aloud to the group along with you. In addition, she can play the drum and count aloud the eight beats of the transition. She can also think of different loco-motor movements for the last part of the activity.

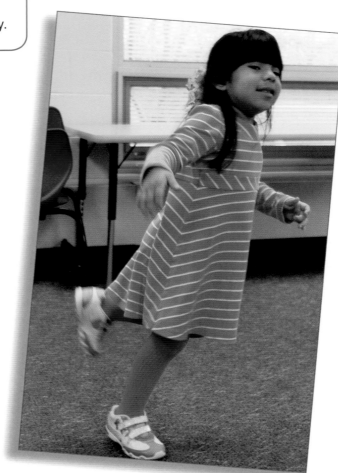

Silly Dance

. . . .

"Silly Dance" is a lively activity using a poem as the prompt. The children will first learn to repeat the poem, then they will learn the movements. Once they have mastered the words and movements, they can perform them together. "Silly Dance" ends with the children dancing freely throughout the space.

What You Need

☼ a small space (the free dance at the end of the activity can be done moving throughout the shared space)

☼ "Kweezletown" instrumental (disc 2, track 27)

What You Do

For this activity, the children can stand in a circle or in home spots throughout the room. Begin by reciting this poem to the children:

Silly Dance

Let's all do a silly dance.
Jump and turn and stomp and prance!
Hop around the hill of ants.
Row your boat all the way to France!
Arms move your shirt and legs move your pants.
Make a funny face and that's our dance!

Now the children will dance to the poem. The poem itself serves as the movement prompt, so say the words slowly and pause whenever necessary

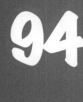

to allow the children to fulfill their movement ideas. Teach the movements that accompany the words:

Let's all do a silly dance.

- shake your whole body—arms, legs, head, torso

Jump and turn and stomp and prance!

- jump up and down once, turn around quickly in place, stomp once or twice, and prance lightly several times; say this line especially slowly, giving the children time to do all the movements—it is not necessary to move exactly in sync with the words

Hop around the hill of ants.

- make a small circular pattern around your home spot while hopping, then do it in the opposite direction; say this line slowly, too, or pause after saying it, to give the children time to do the movement

Row your boat all the way to France!

- squat low and row with both arms

Arms move your shirt [pause] **and legs move your pants.**

- first move arms as many ways as possible, then do the same with legs

Make a funny face and that's our dance!

- make a funny face and silly shape with the body as an ending position

Now put the two together. You say the words, and the children can join you in saying them once they have learned them, doing the movements in response to the words. Be sure to say the poem slowly when you perform the words and movements at the same time (especially lines two and three), and pause after each line. That way there is time to complete the movements before moving on to a new line.

At the end of the activity, have the children take a silly bow. Say to the children:

How can you take a bow and make it silly for the ending of the "Silly Dance"?

To expand the activity, play "Kweezletown" instrumental. Prompt the children to do a silly dance to the music freely in the space, using movement ideas from the poem, and finish with a silly bow.

Modifications

Invite the child to help you call out the words of the poem while the others are moving. Quietly prompt him with the words before you say each line, and then have him repeat them aloud to the group with you.

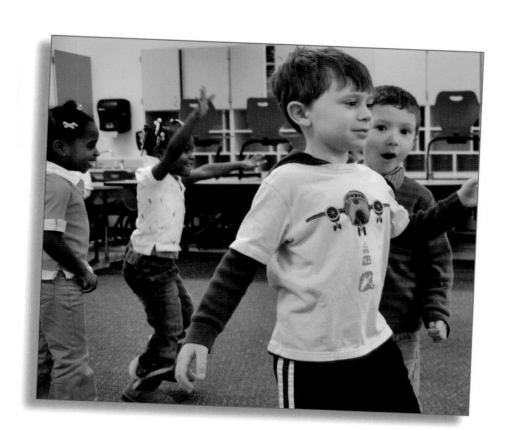

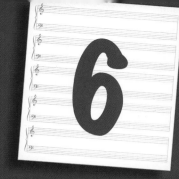

QUIET DOWN AND SAY GOOD-BYE

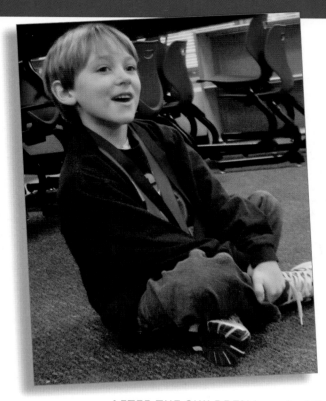

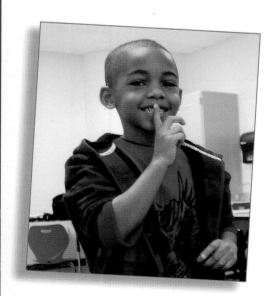

AFTER THE CHILDREN have had the opportunity to participate in a lively physical activity, it is helpful to bring them back to a restful state, ready for the next part of the day or for saying good-bye at the end of the day. "Quiet Down and Say Good-Bye" presents ideas for calming and quieting children after an energetic activity or at the end of the day. Some of the movement ideas are very short, while some are longer, with dramatic play and story dances included. Choose one when you would like to help the children transition into feeling calmer and more relaxed.

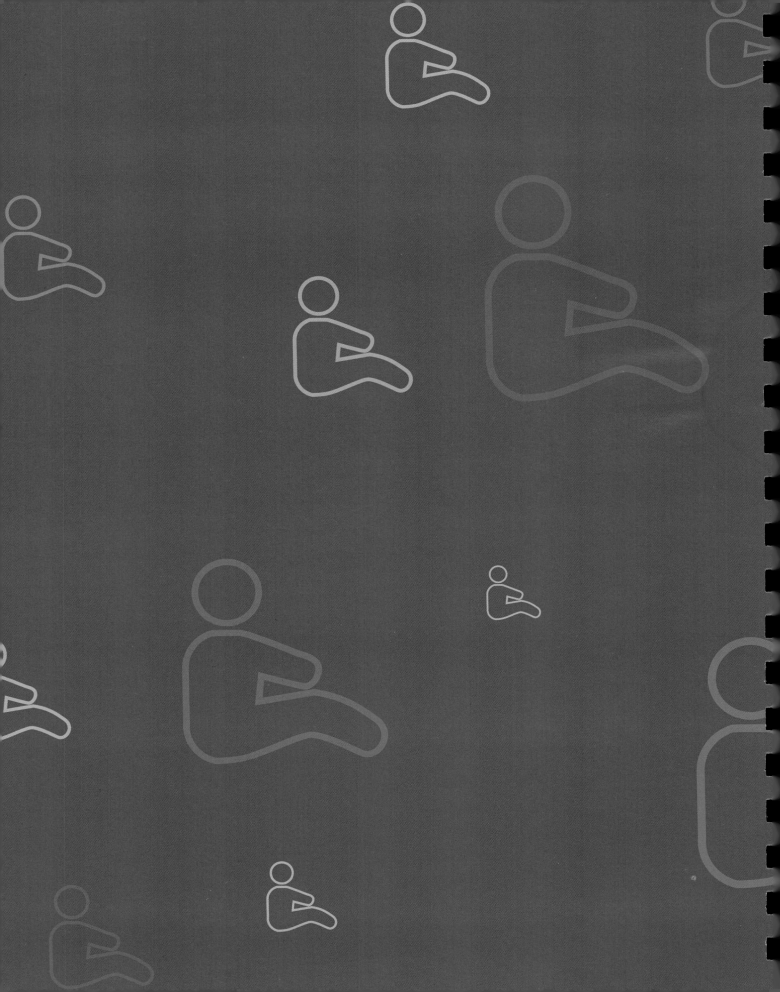

How Can We Bow?

A bow or curtsy is the traditional signal to an audience that a performance has come to an end. Performers bow as a way of acknowledging and thanking the audience. A symbolic movement that is done as a closing gesture, a bow is a fitting finish to any movement session.

What You Need

☼ a small space

What You Do

A bow (bending forward at the waist) or curtsy (doing the same movement but with one leg bent behind) is a basic movement gesture. Make it part of a creative exercise by correlating it to a theme or movement idea from another activity. For example:

- for Activity 68: Dance Story—Dinosaur Romp, say to the children:

Let's finish our dinosaur free dance by thinking about how a dinosaur would bow. What dinosaurs have we danced about today? How about a brontosaurus bow? What about a pterodactyl? Bow like a pterodactyl with its great big wings! How would a tyrannosaurus bow?

- for Activity 24: Space Suits and Activity 75: Grocery Space Trip, say to the children:

Wouldn't it be difficult to bow if you were wearing a great big space suit? Let's try it!

- for Activities 33–50: Action Alphabet, say to the children:

95

Can you make yourself into the shape of the letter and try to bow while holding your letter shape?

• for Activity 70: Eating Healthy, say to the children:

Can you bow in the shape of your favorite fruit or vegetable?

Referring to these examples as guides, use the bow at the end of any session as a way to put a period or exclamation point on the activity. You can ask the children to bow to you one by one, to turn and bow to the child on either side, or to bow all together one more time.

To calm and quiet them after a lively movement session, such as Activity 76: Dancing Statues, you could say to the children:

Let's line up and take a bow. After I point to you one by one, I would like you to take the shape of one of the statues today, and imagine how that statue would bow. Next take the shape of another statue, and bow in that shape to your neighbor on each side. Face me, take your favorite statue shape, and we will do one last bow all together!

Modifications

Because this activity is very open ended, each child can think of a bow that he can do based on his abilities. For example, if a child cannot stand, he can perform a bow from a seated or kneeling position.

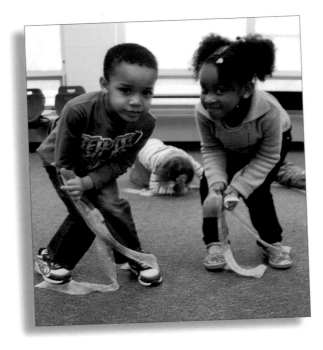

Return to the Nest

This activity is similar to the finish for Activity 66: Dance Story—Baby Birdie Boogie. It can be used as a way to quiet children down after a movement session or simply as a way to gather the children together any time of the day.

What You Need

☼ a small space

☼ "Little Birdie" (disc 1, track 9)

What You Do

Begin the activity with the children standing in a home spot, spread throughout the space. Play "Little Birdie." Say to the children:

Baby birdies, it's time now for you to rest. Let's fly from your home spots to the nest. The nest is the place where we meet for our circle. Fly home to the nest! Let's gather here as all the baby birdies come flying, one by one, to make a soft landing in the nest.

Do you hear the words in the song? The song talks about taking a rest in the nest.

Now that we are all together in the nest, let's listen to the song one more time. We will sway from side to side as we listen to the restful, quiet words in the song.

Modifications

A child who is unable to participate in the larger movement portions (flying and landing) can begin sitting in the nest and stay there throughout the activity.

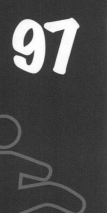

97

Slow-Motion Wave

This is a brief and quiet activity and a good way for the children to say good-bye to you and each other at the end of the day. The challenge of moving in slow motion helps children develop body control while calming down. You can make it more fun by prompting the children to smile, laugh, and blink in slow motion while they are waving.

Modifications

The body parts for waving can be chosen according to the unique needs of the children. If a child is very limited in her movement, she can blink her eyes or flutter her fingers for her good-bye wave.

What You Need

☼ **a small space**

What You Do

Have the children sit in a circle. Say to them:

It is time to say good-bye. As we sit in a circle together, we will wave good-bye with our hands. With one hand, wave good-bye to someone next to you. Then wave to the person on your other side. Now switch hands, and wave to someone across the circle from you. Wave good-bye to everyone else with both hands!

Now let's think of another part of the body that we can wave. We will wave good-bye with our feet! We will wave just like we did with our hands, but now we will do it with our feet, and in slow motion. Can you wave your foot—very slowly—first to the person next to you, then to the person on the other side of you, and to the person across the circle, and to everyone else? Remember, we are waving in slow motion! Let's do all those waves with the other foot. Now wave to as many people as you can with both feet at the same time, still in slow motion!

Let's do the same thing with all of the other parts of our body that can wave (suggest eyes, head, shoulders, elbows, upper body, knees, legs), **and let's continue to do it in slow motion.**

Let's finish by waving all of the body parts together in slow motion!

Floating Balloons

The first part of "Floating Balloons" is somewhat active, but the pace of the activity gradually slows, and at the end, the children finish the session quietly. "Floating Balloons" may become a favorite finishing activity and can be repeated often.

What You Need

- ☼ a large space
- ☼ "Pelican" instrumental (disc 2, track 34)

What You Do

Modifications

A child who is unable to move around can sit or lie down and imagine she is a balloon and move her arms and legs in response to the movement prompts.

The script below contains many movement prompts, so allow the children time to develop each idea before you move on to the next one. Start by asking them to gather around you, standing in a loose group. Say to the children:

Let's imagine we are all balloons. What color balloon would you like to be today? What shape is your balloon? How big is it?

We are light, bright balloons floating in the sky. Doesn't it feel wonderful to be sailing through the sky? What do you see around you? What do you see way down below? Look how high we are! Can you turn softly with the breeze? Can you swoop down low and float up high? Soar through the clouds! What does that feel like?

Our balloons are beginning to lose air. We will move more and more slowly now, and gently drift toward the ground. We have landed back on the ground. Stop in a spot where no one else is, and finish your slow-motion fall until you are lying on the floor—a flat balloon that has lost all of its air!

99

Quiet Stretches and Peaceful Breathing

• • • • • • • • • • • • • • •

Intentional quiet breathing and gentle stretching can have an immediate calming effect on children. "Quiet Stretches and Peaceful Breathing" is especially effective after the children have had the opportunity to be active and are ready to take a rest. You can also use it to finish out the day on a quiet note.

What You Need

☼ a small space

What You Do

The children should begin seated in a circle. Sit with them in the circle so they can see and follow you. Say to them:

Let's cross our legs and stretch our arms to the sky. Now reach your arms out to the side, and then bring them down slowly so they touch the floor next to you. Turn your head to the side, and then to the other side, and look up, and then down, and then back to the center, where you started. Move your shoulders up and down, and circle them forward, then back.

Take a deep breath through your nose. As you let the breath out through your mouth, lower your head. Then take your upper body slowly forward, putting your hands on the floor by your sides, to support your upper body. Relax in this forward position, letting your hands on the floor help support your weight as you relax. Slowly roll back up to your sitting position as you inhale again through your nose. Exhale as you slowly curve your body forward again. Repeat this several times.

Let's go forward one more time, and this time, hold the position at the bottom of the curve. Breathe in and out a few times. From here, let your body slowly roll over onto your side and then onto your back.

Bend your knees and put your feet flat on the floor. Close your eyes. Imagine a beautiful ocean, with its waves gently hitting the shore, and then imagine the waves going out, back in, out, and back in to shore. Put your hands on your stomach. Feel your stomach rise and fall with the rhythm of your breathing.

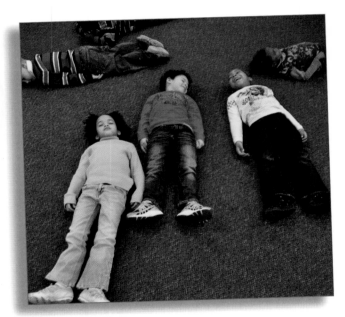

Modifications

A child can participate in the guided relaxing and breathing from a reclining position (lying on his back or side) if sitting is difficult for him.

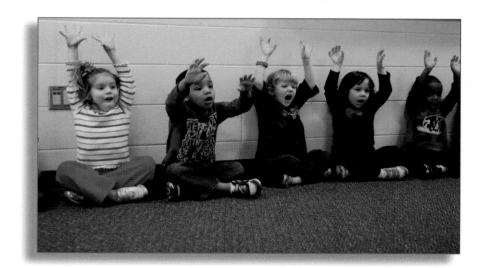

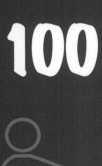

100

Pass Around the Good-Bye

• • • • • • • • • • •

"Pass Around the Good-Bye" is similar to Activity 21: Pass the Movement. It is, however, a quieter activity with smaller movements and does not evolve into a lively dance, so it works well to calm children after more energetic activities, as well as at the end of the day.

What You Need

☼ a small space

What You Do

Have the children sit in circle. Say to them:

I'm going to think of a movement to pass around. We'll use small movements with our upper bodies, arms, hands, and fingers. I will start, and we will all do my movement, one by one, around the circle. Then each of you will have a turn to pick a movement.

Choose a simple movement, such as flapping your elbows or putting your two hands together and giving yourself a handshake. The child next to you will repeat your movement, as will each child in turn. Once the movement has traveled all the way around the circle, the child sitting next to you will think of a movement, and that movement idea will be passed around the circle. When everyone has taken a turn suggesting a movement to pass around, finish by asking the group to do a special good-bye movement together. Here are a few suggestions:

- **Let's each repeat the movement we each created—all at the same time. Let's repeat it a few times all together and try to find a way to stand up while doing the movement.**

- Let's hold hands and pass a gentle squeeze around the circle. When the gentle squeeze comes all the way around, let's let go of our hands, put them up in the air, wave, and say good-bye.

- Let's make a pile of hands. Everyone take several scoots forward, so our circle is smaller and we're sitting closer together. I'll put my hand in, and then, one by one, each of you will put one of your hands on top of mine. We'll do this around the circle, until we have a large stack of hands. Then let's count to three, say good-bye, and lift our hands off the stack.

Modifications

If a child is blind or visually impaired, help him join in the movements by assisting him with each one. For example, with the first movement—flapping elbows—assist him in making his arms into wings, then moving his elbows up and down.

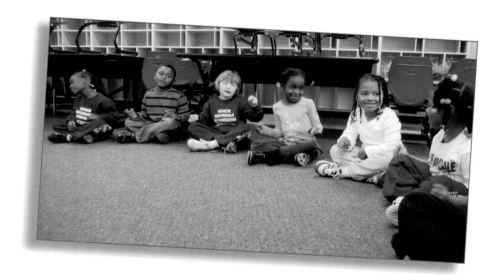

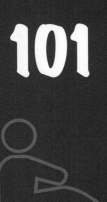

101

Sun Is Setting

· · · · · · · · · · ·

"Sun Is Setting" is similar to Activity 6: Sun Is Rising, a greeting activity. The movements are the same, but the words in the rhyme are different, so it becomes an appropriate finishing or good-bye activity.

What You Need

☼ a small space

What You Do

Have the children sit in a circle. Read the poem to them, and ask them to do the movements corresponding to each line.

Sun is setting, going down.

- sit with crossed legs and make a circle with arms in front of the body, about chest-high

Lights come up all over town.

- lift arms in circle overhead

Moon is rising, feel its glow.

- open arms to the side with palms up, tilt the face up, and close eyes

Night is falling, soft and low.

- return to sitting straight and looking forward as arms float down to floor by sides of legs

Repeat this several times.

Modifications

Children may sit on chairs or in wheelchairs or stand for this activity. For children who are hearing impaired or deaf, draw a picture in four parts, and point them out as you teach the movements: (1) a setting sun, (2) a city at night, (3) a moon, and (4) another picture that depicts nighttime.

Dance Story—
Good Night, Animals!
¡Buenas Noches, Animales!

This short dance story is based on the book *Good Night, Gorilla,* and its Spanish version, *Buenas Noches, Gorila,* by Peggy Rathmann. The author tells a delightful story with very few words—the only written dialogue is "good night," said by the different characters to each other, so the dance story is easy to do in English or Spanish.

What You Need

☼ a large space

☼ "Pelican" instrumental (disc 2, track 34)

☼ *Good Night, Gorilla* or *Buenas Noches, Gorila* by Peggy Rathmann

What You Do

Play "Pelican" instrumental very quietly in the background and read the book to the children. Ask the children to find home spots throughout the space. Play the music again. Say to the children:

Now we will dance the story! I am going to choose Joshua to be the zookeeper, and Mia to be the zookeeper's wife. You can play either role as well. **Mia's home spot will be in the center of the room, in the "house." I would like each of you to think of what animal you would like to be for our dance story. It can be one from the book, or any animal you wish.**

Now, Joshua, you begin walking around, and say good night to each "animal." After you say good night to the first animal, that animal will

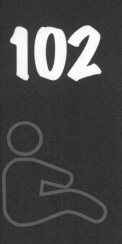

sneak to the house in the center of the room, and silently sit down next to Mia, the zookeeper's wife. When all the animals have snuck over to the house, the zookeeper will then join them. Once we are all together in the circle, we will say good night to each other, and then Mia will lead us each back to our home spot. Mia will then return to the house in the center to join Joshua.

After Mia returns to the house with Joshua, I would like all the animals to sneak back to the house one more time, all together, very quietly! Once you are there, say good night to each other one more time.

Now let's lie down and imagine we are going to sleep. Slowly fade out the music.

Repeat the activity, giving children the chance to try out the different roles.

Modifications

A child who is unable to do the walking part of this activity can sit, stand, or lie down in the area of the house and still be an active participant in the dance story.

Campfire

103

Children will enjoy this activity about going on an imaginary camping trip. It starts out rather lively and has a calm, quiet finish.

What You Need

☼ a small space

What You Do

Begin with the children seated in a circle. Say to them:

Have you ever been camping or hiking in the woods? Have you sat around a campfire? Let's imagine we are spending the night out in the woods. It is time to build a campfire so we can get warm! We will build it in the center of our circle.

First, let's gather wood. Look all around to find pieces that are just right. We need small ones for kindling to get the fire going, and we need bigger ones to keep the fire glowing. Gather as much wood as you can. Let's stack it all up here. Wow, we have quite a pile of wood, don't we!

Now let's put the small pieces in for the beginning of our campfire. Stand back, I am going to light it. We have a wonderful fire. Let's all sit around it in a circle. Don't get too close! Let's warm up our hands, our feet, and feel the warm glow from the fire. I will put a great big log on it so it will keep us warm for a long time.

Now let's all lie back and climb into our sleeping bags. Look up at the sky. What do you see? Let's be very quiet and listen to the sounds of the woods at night. What do you hear?

Modifications

If a child is unable to move around the room to gather wood, put her in charge of helping you to build the imaginary campfire. She can stack the wood that the other children bring and help you build the campfire.

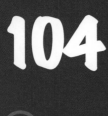

104

Relax from Head to Toe

· · · · · · · · · · · ·

This is a meditative, relaxing exercise. It can be used at the end of an activity, or throughout the day as a break or transition. It also works well as a quiet finish to the day.

What You Need

☼ a small space

☼ "New Baby" instrumental (disc 2, track 32)

☼ small mats (if the floor is not carpeted)

What You Do

Ask the children to go to a spot on the floor where they are not too close to anyone else and lie down. Play "New Baby" instrumental softly in the background.

Let's all relax together. Start by closing your eyes, and think of a place that is relaxing and peaceful, like floating on a raft in a pool, stretching out on the grass looking up at the clouds, or pretending it is night and gazing at the moon and stars.

Now we are going to relax different parts of our bodies while we are lying on the floor. Clench your hands into very tight fists. Now, release your fists, open up your hands, and relax the muscles all the way down to your fingertips. We will do that four more times.

Let's try to make our eyes relax! Squeeze them shut very tight and then relax your eyelids and the muscles around your eyes while you keep your eyes closed. Let's do that four more times.

Try squeezing the muscles in your face. What face do you make when you eat a sour lemon or pickle? Make that face! Now let all those muscles in your face relax. Open your mouth just a little bit so you also relax your strong jaw muscles. Let's do that four more times.

Lift your shoulders up near your ears, and then let them go back down. Do that four more times. Now imagine your shoulders melting into the floor. Stretch your arms long as they stay by your sides and then relax them. Do that four times. Make fists with your hands like we did before, and then relax them.

Stretch your legs all the way down to your toes while you keep them on the floor, then relax them. Let's do that four more times. Now squeeze your toes together as if you are trying to make your foot into a fist, and then relax your feet. Do this with both feet at the same time four more times.

Now feel as though your whole body is melting into the floor. Try to relax everything at once as you slowly melt like an ice cube or a candle.

Modifications

If a child has difficulty lying on the floor, he can do the structured exercise while seated.

Once they have achieved a relaxed state, play the music again. This music is very calm with a slow, peaceful rhythm. While the children are listening to the music, guide them to put their hands on their stomachs and feel the rise and fall of their breathing.

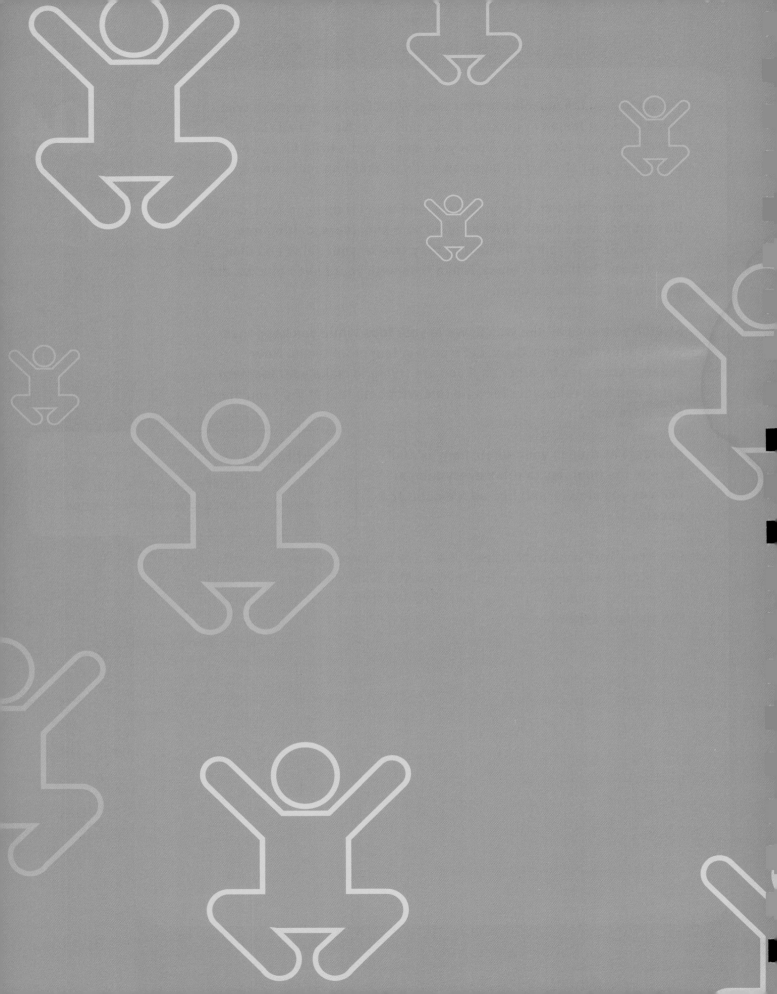

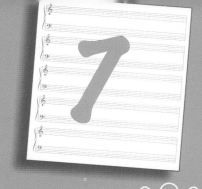

DANCE AND MUSIC PRESENTATION JUMP-STARTS

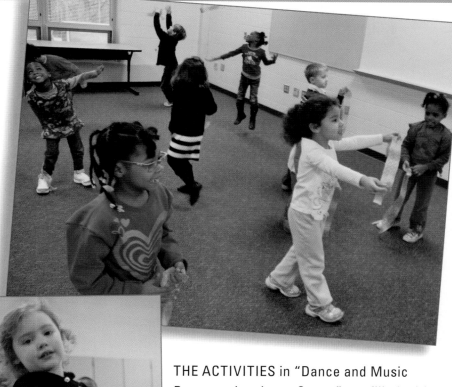

THE ACTIVITIES in "Dance and Music Presentation Jump-Starts" are filled with creative dance ideas that can be used as freestanding movement explorations and as structured presentations for family and friends. The "Presentation Ideas" at the end of each activity will guide you as you prepare for and then lead the children through a performance of the dances. With little extra effort, you will have evolved the movement explorations into fun, enriching experiences for the children—and for the audience! Activity 109: Busy Bugs: A Multilayered Movement Study is designed for use over several days, with instructions for a performance on the last day.

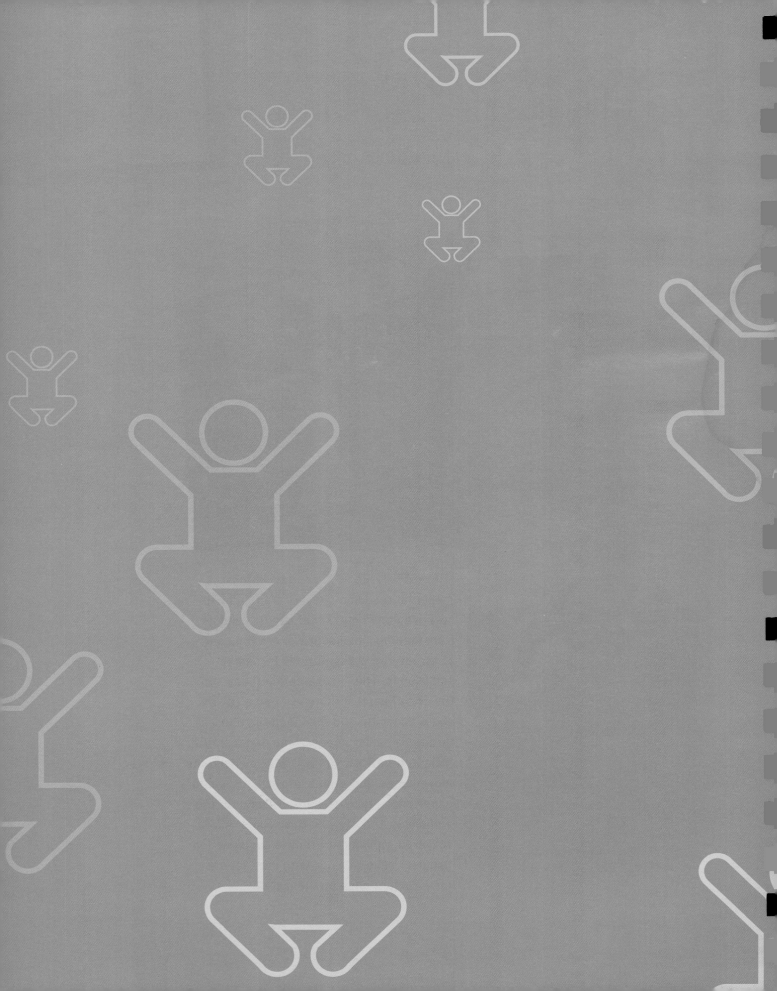

Colors of the Rainbow

This activity is an extended movement study based on the theme of color. It will take about an hour to an hour and a half, including the time it takes to help the children make ribbon bangles. If you expand it into a presentation, plan to add about an extra half hour to hang the large sheet of paper on which you write the children's suggestions in the opening section of the lesson, hang the paper plate rainbows, place the bangle props, get your music set up, and have the children in their spots ready to begin the dance.

What You Need

☼ a large space

☼ "Catsup" instrumental (disc 1, track 17), "Goldie Rock" instrumental (disc 2, track 23), "Care of the Earth" instrumental (disc 1, track 16), and "Shine & Brighten" instrumental (disc 2, track 37)

☼ a large roll of paper; red, yellow, and blue markers; the book *Color Dance* by Ann Jonas; pipe cleaners and precut ten-inch strips of ribbon in many different colors; crayons of many colors; paper plates

What You Do

Begin with the children seated in a circle. These places will be their home spots as you introduce each new color. Say to the children:

Today we are going to dance about all the colors! What is your favorite color? Why is it your favorite color? How does thinking about that color make you feel?

First let's talk about red. Can you think of some things that are red? Let's name as many red things as we can think of, and I will use a red marker to write them all down on this big sheet of paper.

Now let's dance about the color red, how it makes us feel, and all of the red things we just named. You may dance freely in the space during the dance. At the end of the music, stop in the shape of something that is red. Play "Catsup" instrumental.

Return to your home spots in the circle, and now let's talk about yellow. Can you name some things that are yellow? Using my yellow marker this time, I will write down the yellow things you think of below the red items.

Let's dance about all of these yellow things, and how the color yellow makes us feel. Finish in the shape of something yellow. Play "Goldie Rock" instrumental.

Follow the same steps with blue—play "Care of the Earth" instrumental. Then, using the markers and paper, demonstrate to the children how green is a mixture of blue and yellow. Say:

All the rest of the colors—orange, indigo, violet, and everything in between—are made from the first three: red, yellow, and blue. These three colors are called "primary colors," because you can make all of the other colors by mixing them together in different ways.

Staying in the circle, read *Color Dance* by Ann Jonas. Say to the children:

This book shows how the primary colors mix together to make other colors, which the children in the story demonstrate by dancing with colorful scarves. Now let's make some colorful bangles as we prepare to do our own color dance.

The colorful bangles can be used as props to expand the color exploration. The children can use them during the final color dance and to enhance the presentation. Bring ribbons of many different colors, enough for at least five ribbons per bangle. Cut the ribbons into ten-inch strips ahead of time.

With the children still seated in the circle, give each one a pipe cleaner that has been twisted and fastened into a circle (be sure to tuck in any sharp ends) and five or six different-colored ribbons. Help the children tie the ribbons on the pipe cleaner so that they hang together off the bangle. The children will each hold a bangle and manipulate it while they are dancing.

If you use "Colors of the Rainbow" as a presentation, decorate the space and further explore the color theme by making rainbows from paper plates, markers, a hole punch, and yarn. Cut the plates in half so the children can use the shape of the plate as the rainbow, filling it in with many colors of crayons. Give the children time to make their rainbows, and then use them as a backdrop during the presentation. Punch a hole in the top-center of each one, and hang them from the ceiling with yarn. You can also tack them to a wall, if that works better in your space.

Now the children are ready to do the color dance. Tell them to find a home spot on the floor so they are evenly spread throughout the space. Play "Shine & Brighten" instrumental. Say to the children:

When the music begins, let's start dancing! You can move throughout the space and dance about all the color ideas we've explored.

- **Think about all the red, yellow, and blue items we wrote down.**

- **Think about all the colors we can make by mixing the primary colors.**

- **Dance about the book we read, and the children who were mixing the colors in that story.**

- **Look at the rainbows you made that are hanging up around the room, and dance about the rainbows.**

- **Use your colorful bangles and move the ribbons while you dance!**

Finish the "Colors of the Rainbow" dance with the children taking a big bow in a line while shaking their bangles.

Presentation Ideas

The "Colors of the Rainbow" dance makes a colorful and fun presentation for family, friends, and/or fellow students. The presentation can last from fifteen to thirty minutes, depending on how you expand the dance.

Modifications

Because this is an activity that explores color through so many different media, there are numerous opportunities for participation. Some children may be able to respond by doing smaller movements in response to all of the prompts. In addition, a child could hold the paper and markers for you during the first part of the activity. He could hold the book for you as you read it. He could run the music. He could call out prompts such as "Dance about the color red!" and hold and manipulate his prop while the others are dancing.

Hang the large sheet of paper on which you documented all of the children's different color ideas as a background and the paper plate rainbows the children made. Before the children dance, take a few minutes to explain to the audience the explorations that led up to the dance: learning about primary colors, naming objects of those colors, dancing about each color, reading and discussing ideas from the book *Color Dance* (you can show and describe the book), making colorful bangles, and drawing rainbows.

Ask the children to take their places. They can come out as a group, or one by one, to find their home spots. Or the children can already be standing in their home spots. Talk to them ahead of time about how they want to begin the dance so they can contribute to structuring the presentation. Play "Shine & Brighten" instrumental while the children do the color dance. End with the children lined up to take a bow.

To expand the presentation, divide the children into three groups and ask each group to dance about red, yellow, or blue. Play "Catsup," "Goldie Rock," and "Care of the Earth" instrumentals, respectively. After each group has danced about its primary color, have the children do the "Colors of the Rainbow" dance together as a group, using the bangle props. Finish with the children in a line facing the audience, and have them bow while shaking the bangles.

Here are more ideas for expanding and enhancing the presentation:

- Suggest to the children that they wear their favorite color for the presentation.

- If you begin the presentation with the three groups each dancing about a primary color, make a separate set of bangles using ribbons of that color for each group.

- Elicit ideas from the children about how they would like to expand the exploration. For example, you could ask them: "Would you like to do a dance just about your favorite color?" "What kind of music would you like to use for that dance?" Offer a selection from the list of thirty instrumental pieces included on the CDs that accompany this book. Incorporate the children's ideas into the presentation.

Dance Story—
The Sun Is My Favorite Star

Bringing a story alive through dance and music enhances reading comprehension and reinforce sequencing as the children learn the order of the story by exploring each section through movement. In addition, dance stories give children a new way to express and dramatize events and characters in a story. There are seven sections to this dance story, based on five movement images from Frank Asch's book *The Sun Is My Favorite Star.*

What You Need

☼ a large space

☼ "Shine & Brighten" instrumental and "Sunscreen" (disc 2, track 37 and disc 1, track 12)

☼ *The Sun Is My Favorite Star* by Frank Asch and sparkly fabric streamers (the streamers can also be used for Activity 108: Dance Story—*The Snowy Day*)

What You Do

Make streamers ahead of time by cutting strips about twelve inches long and three inches wide from inexpensive sparkly fabric. Read *The Sun Is My Favorite Star* to the children. Ask them to find home spots throughout the space to begin the dance story. Play "Shine & Brighten" instrumental. Allow each section of the dance to develop as the children choose how they want to react to the story, music, movement prompts, and props. Say to them:

Let's all lie down and close our eyes so we can begin our dance by waking up, like the child in the book. Wake up, it's morning; the sunlight is coming in the window! Time to get dressed and have breakfast.

Now it's time to go out and play. On a beautiful, sunny day, what do you like to do outside? Play on the playground? Play ball and other games with your friends? Imagine you are swinging from a tire in a tree, like the picture in the book, and then pull the little red wagon.

Run in and out of the trees as the sun follows you. Now imagine you are the sun, and play hide-and-seek in the clouds. Shine your bright rays on the Earth.

It's raining! Feel the rain on your face. Swirl and fall like the raindrops.

Imagine a beautiful rainbow. Try to reach it! Can you jump up and touch it? Run under it, around it, run from one end of it to the other, and jump over it! What if you could climb up one side and slide down the other?

Imagine you have a crayon, and draw the beautiful sunset. Try to fill the whole space, reaching high and low, and draw your picture in the air.

Now dance freely about all the fun ideas in this story and anything else about the sun that makes you want to dance! Play "Sunscreen" and pass out the sparkly streamers.

Allow the children to decide how they want to start and finish the dance. You can ask, "Should we enter from the side and each walk to a home spot in the space?" or "Should we finish in a shape from the story?"

This activity can be adapted to a smaller space by having each child move within a home spot. Or divide the group up so one group is moving and the other group or groups are participating as audience. Give a task to the group that is the audience, saying, for example, "What games do you see the children pretending to play outside?"

Presentation Ideas

"Dance Story—*The Sun Is My Favorite Star*" will be a short, informal presentation about fifteen minutes long for family, friends, and/or fellow students. Explain to the audience that there are two parts to the dance story and that the children have explored movement ideas from the book *The Sun Is My Favorite Star*. Place the streamers just to the side of the performance area so the children can easily retrieve them for the second part of the dance.

Have the children ready to enter the space from the side, or have them already standing in their home spots. Play "Shine & Brighten" instrumental and prompt the children to go through their movement ideas as you read the story slowly, just as before. They will begin by waking up and finish by drawing the sunset in the air.

For the second part, ask the children to pick up their streamers and take their places to start the free dance. Play "Sunscreen" instrumental and prompt the children to manipulate their streamers and dance throughout the space. Finish the dance with an ending previously agreed upon by the children.

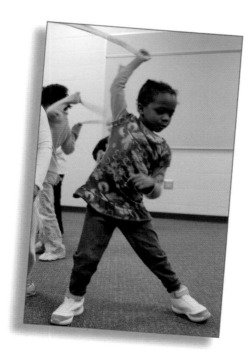

Modifications

One of the advantages of a dance story is that children may participate as much or as little as they are able and willing. Once everyone is familiar with the story, there are many different opportunities to participate in this movement activity. A child who has difficulty participating in the large-movement portions of this activity can join with the other children by doing smaller movements in response to the prompts. For example, she may choose to dance the part of the sun in the story, which can be done in a stationary spot with little movement. She can hold and manipulate the streamer, draw with an imaginary crayon in the space around her, and she can help you call out the prompts: "It's raining! Feel the rain on your face!" She can also sing along to the words of "Sunscreen" while the others are dancing.

Dance Story—Pumpkin Patch

· · · · · · · · · · ·

"Pumpkin Patch" is a story about a visit to the pumpkin patch. The children will improvise a dance while you tell the story. It is based on an autumn theme, but the ideas in the story will spark the children's imaginations any time of the year.

What You Need

- ☼ a small space
- ☼ "Monster Spray" instrumental (disc 2, track 31)
- ☼ small flashlights (optional)

What You Do

If you have them, pass out small flashlights and turn off the room lights if this works in your space. Ask the children to gather behind you in a loosely structured group. Play "Monster Spray" instrumental quietly in the background. Be sure to allow time for the children to develop each movement prompt. Say to them:

Let's go to the pumpkin patch! We'll walk across the fields until we get there.

Here we are! Now explore the patch and search for the perfect pumpkin. Let's take very high steps so we don't trip over all the pumpkin vines. It's getting dark. Look! We have a beautiful full moon to light our way. Do you see the moon and sparkly stars in the sky on this cool, clear night?

Bend over and look at each pumpkin closely. Have you found a pumpkin you like? Pick it up! Let's carry our pumpkins back home. Uh-oh! We've picked out the biggest ones, and they are so heavy. Can we carry them?

How does it make you walk when you have something so heavy to carry? Let's keep going. You can do it! Use your flashlight to help you see the way.

Look, I see a light on in the house over there. We are almost home! Let's try to hurry home with our heavy pumpkins.

Now we are home, and we can carve our pumpkins. What face will you put on yours? A happy one? A scary one? Sit down in a circle, and let's try out some faces on ourselves first. Make a happy face, silly face, scary face, shy face. Which one do you like best? Imagine you are carving your pumpkin with the expression you like best.

Now I will play the music again, and you can dance about our visit to the pumpkin patch. Think about going through the field, the moon and stars, all the pumpkins, searching for and picking out your pumpkins, carrying the heavy pumpkins home, carving them, and making lots of different faces. You may use your flashlights during this dance, and you can leave the circle and dance freely throughout the space. When the music stops, finish in the shape of a pumpkin! Play "Monster Spray" instrumental.

Presentation Ideas

"Pumpkin Patch" makes a fun, short presentation. When doing the dance for an audience, follow the same steps as above. Tell the audience the story of the trip to the pumpkin patch, and as you do, the children will respond to the prompts. Play "Monster Spray" instrumental softly in the background.

Finish with the children carving an imaginary pumpkin face when the music ends. Then ask them to dance freely to the music (play "Monster Spray" instrumental again, this time at normal volume) using all the ideas from the visit to the pumpkin patch and finishing the dance in the shape of a pumpkin. To end the presentation, have the children bow to the audience. Prompt the children by asking them, "How would a great big round pumpkin do a bow?"

Modifications

A child who has difficulty participating in the movement portions of this activity can do smaller movements in response to the prompts. For example, she can look up and imagine the moon and stars, hold and manipulate a flashlight, make faces along with the other children, pretend to carve a pumpkin, and take a bow. For the presentation, she can help you call out the story. You say the phrases quietly to her first and then she calls them out to the children: "Take high steps through the pumpkin patch!"

108

Dance Story— The Snowy Day

· · · · · · · · · · · ·

Bringing a story alive through dance and music is a way to enhance reading comprehension and reinforce sequencing, as the children learn the order of the story by exploring each section through movement. In addition, dance stories give children a new way to express and dramatize the events and characters in a story. There are five sections to this dance story, based on five movement images from the book *The Snowy Day* by Ezra Jack Keats. Dancing about these images will bring the story to life for the children.

What You Need

☼ a large space

☼ "Snow People" instrumental and "Snowy Owl" instrumental (disc 2, tracks 38 and 39)

☼ *The Snowy Day* by Ezra Jack Keats and strips of white mesh or netting fabric or sparkly fabric streamers (optional) (the streamers can also be used for Activity 106: Dance Story—*The Sun Is My Favorite Star*)

What You Do

Make small mesh or netting fabric snowflakes (tie two six-inch strips of white mesh or fabric netting together) or make streamers by cutting strips about twelve inches long and three inches wide from inexpensive sparkly fabric (optional). Read *The Snowy Day* aloud. Play "Snow People" instrumental quietly. Ask the children to sit in their home spots spread throughout the large space and say to them:

Let's dance the story! Imagine you are cuddled up in your warm bed. Wake up, yawn, rub your eyes, and stretch your arms, your hands, your legs, your feet, your whole body, while sitting in bed. Stand up, stretch your whole body again, go to the window, open the curtains, and look outside. What do you see?

Don't you want to go out and play in that beautiful snow? Put on your snowsuits, boots, mittens, hats, scarves. Let's go out in the snow!

Let's try to walk through the snow: First walk, then trudge, stomp, tiptoe, point your toes in, point your toes out, create walking patterns in the snow, walk backward, drag your feet in the snow, play follow the leader! Remember to give the children time to explore each new idea.

Now let's play in the snow some more: roll snowballs; build a snow-person, then melt; make snow angels; make your body into snowflake shapes; jump over a snow bank; twirl like the swirling snow; ice-skate; go for a sled ride; sit and spin in a snow saucer. Pretend to climb up a mountain like the little boy in the book, and then slide all the way down!

I will play some different music (play "Snowy Owl" instrumental), **and you can dance about our day in the snow again. We will dance freely in the large space about all of the ideas we just had!**

If you have them, pass out the fabric snowflakes or sparkly streamers for this free dance. Encourage the children to find new and interesting ways to use them. If the children are using fabric snowflakes, say:

Can you throw your snowflake in the air and catch it? Let's do that all together to create a snow flurry!

If the children are using sparkly streamers, say:

Can you move them slowly? Quickly? Can you move them up and down? Can you twirl them as you turn like swirling snow?

Finish the dance by telling the children to make their bodies into snow-flake shapes and hold the shapes.

This activity can be adapted to a smaller space, with children moving around their home spots. You can also divide the children so that one group dances while the other becomes the audience. Give the audience group a task by saying to them, for example, "How many snowflake shapes did you see?"

Presentation Ideas

"Dance Story—*The Snowy Day*" makes a fun, short presentation. Perform all of the steps of the activity for an audience. First read the book, then tell the story of the day in the snow as the children respond to the prompts. Play "Snow People" instrumental softly in the background. Then ask the children to dance freely with the props to "Snowy Owl" instrumental, played at normal volume. Ask the children to think about all the ideas from the book and from the movement prompts.

Modifications

One of the advantages of a dance story is that children may participate as much or as little as they are able and willing. A child who is unable to participate in the large-movement portions of this activity can participate with the other children by doing smaller movements in response to the prompts. For example, she can imagine she is waking up, stretching, looking out the window, dressing in snow gear, and whatever other movements she can do in response to the story. She can also hold and manipulate a streamer or snowflake prop. For the presentation, she can help you tell the story. You say the phrases quietly to her first, and then she calls them out to the children: "Make footprints in the snow!"

Finish the dance by asking the children to make a snowflake shape or a shape from another idea in the story. You and the children may want to end the presentation with a bow. Ask the children, "How would a great big round snowperson do a bow? What if he then quickly melted to the ground?"

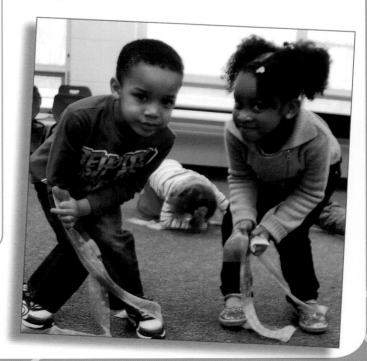

Busy Bugs: A Multilayered Movement Study

"Busy Bugs: A Multilayered Movement Study" is an activity about insects divided into five sessions. It can be developed over five consecutive days (which is how it is presented here) or each session can be done on its own, as a supplement to another lesson, or as part of a story about insects. Each of the five sessions has the same warm-up and large-motor skills practice, which begins with the children seated in a circle and progresses to the children standing and moving across the floor. You can add any ideas or variations you and the children develop as you repeat the warm-up and large-motor skills exercises.

The five Busy Bug movement sessions are:

- Session 1—Silly Spiders

- Session 2—Moths and Butterflies

- Session 3—Squeegy Bugs

- Session 4—So Many Bugs!

- Session 5—Dancing about Bugs for Parents and Friends

The sessions contain free dance activities, each with unique variations, including stories, pictures, and props. The fourth session, "So Many Bugs!" has the children creating antennae to wear for the informal performance with an audience on the last day. The sessions are each structured to last about an hour, but time spent will vary depending on how long the transitions between sections take, and how much you allow the different sections to develop as you and the children add your own ideas. The informal performance on the last day is a culmination of the explorations in the first four sessions. The fifth session lasts approximately an hour to an hour and a half, including preparation time; the actual performance takes about a half-hour.

If you use all five sessions of this activity consecutively, remind the children from time to time during the first four sessions that they will be showing their dances and drawings to an audience at the end of the week. Invite family, friends, and/or fellow students to attend the performance on the last day. The number of people you invite will of course depend on the size of your space. Be sure to allow enough room for the children to do the movement explorations with the audience seated facing them.

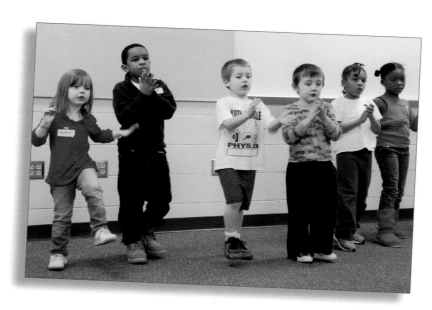

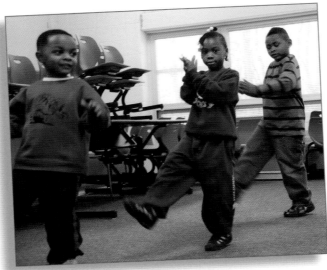

Busy Bugs
Session 1: Silly Spiders

The characteristics and behavior of spiders provide the inspiration for the movement activities in "Busy Bugs Session 1: Silly Spiders." In addition to a warm-up and large-motor skills practice, this session contains a rhythm pattern activity, a silly spider art project, and free dance.

What You Need

☼ a large space

☼ "Calamity Sam" instrumental (disc 1, track 15)

☼ a long roll of white paper; crayons; pictures of unusual spiders; a drum or a tambourine

What You Do

Begin with a warm-up about different kinds of bugs and how they move. Add ideas and variations you and the children develop as you do the warm-up. Start by asking the children to sit in a circle.

Warm-Up

Say to the children:

We will use ideas from the world of insects for our warm-up!

- **While you are sitting, curl in and out like a pill bug. Try it lying down.**

- **Roll onto your back, and imagine you are a bug that is stuck on its back. Move your arms and legs as many ways as you can.**

- Roll from side to side like a roly-poly bug, and then bring yourself back up to sitting.

- Inch around the circle like a caterpillar, and end up back where you started.

- Imagine you are a spider, going up and down on your silver thread. Go up and down again, up and down, and finish standing up.

- Let's imagine we are little crickets, and do small bounces as we bend our knees and then straighten them. Now let's take off from the floor as we do little bouncy jumps.

Large-Motor Skills Practice

Now say to the children:

We are warmed up and ready to do some larger movements across the floor! Let's make a line across the floor, so we can go back and forth while we practice the bigger movements.

As they respond to your movement prompts, the children will travel across the floor together, lined up side by side, with plenty of room between them, and then come back across. Use a drum or tambourine to keep the beat.

- **Let's march all the way across the floor together, marching like hard-working ants! Do the same thing coming back across.**

- **Let's tiptoe like a very quiet bug, all the way across and all the way back.**

- **Let's hop and jump like a grasshopper as it goes from one blade of grass to another, all the way across a field.**

- **Let's run and swoop like a moth as it flies around a bright light at night. Remember to slow down as you get close to the other side.**

- **Let's skip like a water bug across a pond.** Skips are for children ages five and up.

- **Let's leap like a butterfly taking off and landing.** Leaps are for children ages five and up.

Rhythm Pattern Game

The next section of the activity is a rhythm exercise and an excellent movement game that hones listening and understanding skills. The children will listen for and interpret your rhythm cues and then respond with the appropriate movements. Say to the children:

Everyone find a home spot. We are going to play a rhythm game. Some of you are going to be grasshoppers, some butterflies, and some are going to be pill bugs. Everyone will have a turn to be each insect. Divide the children into three groups.

The grasshoppers will jump three times when they hear me beat the tambourine three times sharply. Butterflies will lift their arms and lower them when they hear the soft shaking of the tambourine. Pill bugs will curl in and out, standing, sitting, or lying on the floor, when I tap the tambourine softly twice.

Randomly play the rhythms several times—three sharp beats, a few moments of soft shaking, two soft taps—while the appropriate group responds. After a few repetitions, change groups so that each child gets the chance to be a grasshopper, a butterfly, and a pill bug.

Draw a Silly Spider

Bring the children together seated in a circle and show them pictures of unusual spiders. Say to the children:

Let's take a rest. I would like you to use your imaginations and think about your own ideas for how a spider might look. What would you like it to be? What color? How big? What would its eyes and face look like? Its legs? Its body? What kind of web would it spin? How would it move?

Now you will draw the spider you are imagining! I will roll out this long sheet of paper on the floor and give each of you a place to sit and some crayons so that you can draw your spider.

Make sure each child has plenty of room on the paper, because the children will add more bug drawings to the paper during later sessions.

Free Dance—Silly Spiders

When the children are finished drawing, put the paper aside and ask the children to find home spots throughout the large space. Say:

Let's dance freely about the new spider you created in your imagination and then drew on the paper. When the music finishes, I would like you to move like a spider back to your home spot, and freeze in the shape of your spider to end our dance! Play "Calamity Sam" instrumental.

Presentation Ideas

Busy Bugs Session 1: Silly Spiders becomes part of the informal presentation to be performed by the children on the last day of this five-session Busy Bugs activity. If, however, you want to present ideas from this session as a mini-performance, there are several things that make a fun presentation:

- the warm-up and large-motor skills practice
- the rhythm pattern game
- the silly spiders free dance, using the silly spiders drawing as a backdrop

After the children freeze in their spider shapes at the end of the free dance, ask them to end the mini-performance with a silly spider bow.

For more performance tips, review points one through five and also nine in the list on pages 300–302.

Modifications

Have the child who is unable to stand participate in the floor portion of the warm-up. He can help keep the beat by clapping or playing a drum or tambourine during the large-motor skills practice.

For the rhythm pattern activity, modify the movements to fit children's needs. For example, if someone in the grasshopper group is unable to jump, ask her to lift her arms, hands, shoulders, fingers, or toes up and down instead.

The silly spider free dance at the end can be performed in one spot on the floor seated, standing, or lying down, instead of moving through space, to accommodate children who are not ambulatory.

Busy Bugs Session 2: Moths and Butterflies

The activities in "Busy Bugs Session 2: Moths and Butterflies" are built around the life cycle of the moth and butterfly. Children will dance about the life cycle from caterpillar to moth or butterfly, using props to enhance the dance story. This session finishes with a caterpillar conga dance!

What You Need

☼ a large space

☼ "Goldie Waltz" instrumental (disc 2, track 24), "Bumblebee" instrumental (disc 1, track 14), and "Shakers" instrumental (disc 2, track 36)

☼ crayons; pictures of or a book about the life cycle of a moth or butterfly; a black cloth large enough for all the children to fit under when clustered together, crouched on the floor (optional); small squares of sparkly fabric (approximately twelve by twelve inches); a drum or a tambourine

What You Do

Begin with a warm-up about different kinds of bugs and how they move. Add ideas and variations you and the children develop as you do the warm-up. Start by asking the children to sit in a circle.

Warm-Up

Say to the children:

We will use ideas from the world of insects for our warm-up!

- **While you are sitting, curl in and out like a pill bug. Try it lying down.**

- **Roll onto your back, and imagine you are a bug that is stuck on its back. Move your arms and legs as many ways as you can.**

- **Roll from side to side like a roly-poly bug, and then bring yourself back up to sitting.**

- **Inch around the circle like a caterpillar, and end up back where you started.**

- **Imagine you are a spider, going up and down on your silver thread. Go up and down again, up and down, and finish standing up.**

- **Let's imagine we are little crickets and do small bounces as we bend our knees and then straighten them. Now let's take off from the floor as we do little bouncy jumps.**

Large-Motor Skills Practice

Now say to the children:

We are warmed up and ready to do some larger movements across the floor! Let's make a line so we can go back and forth while we practice the bigger movements.

As they respond to your movement prompts, the children will travel across the floor together, lined up side by side, with plenty of room between them, and then come back across. Use a drum or tambourine to keep the beat.

- **Let's march all the way across the floor together, marching like hard-working ants! Do the same thing coming back across.**

- **Let's tiptoe like a very quiet bug, all the way across and all the way back.**

- **Let's walk fast in a zigzag pattern like a spider, all the way across and all the way back.**

- **Let's hop and jump like a grasshopper as it goes from one blade of grass to another, all the way across a field.**

- **Let's run and swoop like a moth as it flies around a bright light at night. Remember to slow down as you get close to the other side.**

- **Let's skip like a water bug across a pond.** Skips are for children ages five and up.

- **Let's leap like a butterfly taking off and landing.** Leaps are for children ages five and up.

Dance Story—Caterpillars and Cocoons

In this dance story, the children will dance about the life cycle of a moth or butterfly. Bring the children together to sit in a circle, and show them pictures of the various stages in the moth or butterfly life cycle. The children will interpret the ideas about the cycle in movement. Be sure to allow each section of the dance story to develop as the children respond to your movement prompts. Say to them:

Now we will do a dance about a caterpillar that turns into a moth or butterfly. Before we begin, think about what kind of caterpillar you want to be and what kind of moth or butterfly you will turn into when you emerge from your cocoon.

Go to your home spot. I'm going to play some music, and you can move around the room like little caterpillars. Play "Goldie Waltz" instrumental. **Try to find tasty leaves so you can grow. Do you see some leaves? Inch your way up the tree, and munch on the yummy leaves.**

It's time to spin your cocoon, so you can begin your amazing transformation. Where would you like to spin your cocoon? Find your spot and begin spinning!

If you have a cloth large enough for all the children to fit under, spread it out on the floor now, and ask the children to crawl under it after they have done some spinning. Hold one end of the cloth and assist each child as she crawls under it.

While you're inside the cocoon, transform yourself into a moth or butterfly. When I call your name, come out of the cocoon, and I will give you your wings so you can dance like a moth or butterfly! Give two fabric pieces to each child, and change the music to "Bumblebee" instrumental. **Imagine what it is like to try out your brand new wings!**

Let's finish the dance story with a bow or curtsy. Bow like a butterfly with your new wings!

Draw a Caterpillar, Cocoon, and Moth or Butterfly

Collect the fabric squares. Have the children seat themselves in a circle and say to them:

Now you will draw pictures about the ideas from our dance. I will roll out this long sheet of paper. Please sit down along the edge of the paper while I pass out some crayons. Draw the caterpillar, cocoon, and butterfly or moth you just danced about.

If this project is a continuation from Busy Bugs Session 1, tell the children to find the picture they drew before and draw next to it now.

Caterpillar Conga Line

This is a fun, upbeat movement activity. The children learn the conga rhythm with clapping, then respond to this beat with a variety of movements. (See also Activity 32: Conga Line.) Begin by asking the children to sit in a circle. Say to them:

Now we will finish our life-cycle study by making a giant caterpillar with our bodies. After we learn a new rhythm, everyone will line up behind me. Our legs will become the many legs on a big caterpillar!

The rhythm we're going to learn is a rhythm called the "conga." It has four beats. Clap four times with me: one, two, three, four. This time, we're going to make the fourth beat strong, which is called an accent. One, two three, FOUR! One, two, three, FOUR! This "one-two-three-

FOUR" rhythm is the conga rhythm. Try it with your feet while sitting. Can you move your feet to the rhythm and clap it too? Now stand in place and try the rhythm with your feet: step one, step two, step three, strong-step FOUR.

Repeat this with the children several times. Encourage them to count the rhythm out loud with you while they step in place to the beat.

Now on the strong fourth beat, instead of stepping down onto your foot, stretch your leg to the side and touch your toes to the floor. Still standing in place, try putting it all together: step one, step two, step three, touch-floor-with-toes four. Step one, step two, step three, touch-floor-with-toes four. This step-step-step-touch movement is the conga dance!

Ask the children to stand in a straight line behind you with plenty of space between them.

Let's try the conga dance standing together in a line. Let's start out very slowly. We'll step forward on one, two, and three, and then we'll touch our toes to the side on four. Good! Now we'll try it again, a little faster this time. Walk one, two, three, touch four. Walk one, two, three, touch four. Let's try it again, clapping our hands on that strong fourth beat—just like we did while we were sitting in the circle—at the same time we touch our toes to the side. Try it a little faster!

Play "Shakers" instrumental. Lead the children around and out of the room, and tell them to wave good-bye as they dance.

Presentation Ideas

Busy Bugs Session 2: Moths and Butterflies becomes part of the informal presentation to be performed by the children on the last day of this five-session Busy Bugs activity. If, however, you would like to present ideas from this session as a mini-performance, there are several things that would make a fun presentation:

- the warm-up and large-motor skills practice

- the caterpillars and cocoons dance story, using the children's drawings of caterpillars, cocoons, butterflies, or moths as a backdrop

- the caterpillar conga line

To finish the mini-performance, ask the children to return to the performance space to take a butterfly bow after they wave good-bye during the caterpillar conga dance.

For more performance tips, review points one through six and eight and nine in the list on pages 300–302.

Modifications

Have the child who is unable to stand participate in the floor portion of the warm-up. She can help keep the beat by clapping or playing a drum or tambourine during the large-motor skills practice.

The dance story movement can be modified so that the child stays in one place and does not move around during the various parts of the story. Bring the large cloth to cover the child who is stationary, and give her butterfly wings to use while seated.

A child who is blind or is visually impaired can participate in the caterpillar conga line activity. Once she and the other children have learned the beat and the movements, first by clapping, then stepping in place, have the child stand in front of you and put your hands on her shoulders. (The other children will be lined up behind you.) Gently guide her as she begins to move so you can control her direction and pace.

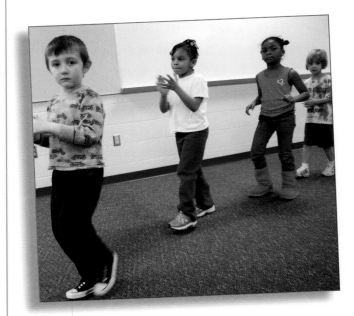

Busy Bugs
Session 3: Squeegy Bugs

109

"Busy Bugs Session 3: Squeegy Bugs," based on the book *The Little Squeegy Bug*, by Bill Martin Jr. and Michael Sampson, is about a bug searching for his identity. During his journey to find out what kind of bug he is, he encounters several other insects and has some new adventures, all of which will be explored by the children through dance and music.

What You Need

☼ a large space

☼ "Monster Spray" instrumental and "Sunscreen" instrumental (disc 2, tracks 31 and 40)

☼ *The Little Squeegy Bug* by Bill Martin Jr. and Michael Sampson; small flashlights or fiber-optic lights; a drum or a tambourine

What You Do

Begin with a warm-up about different kinds of bugs and how they move. Add ideas and variations you and the children develop as you do the warm-up. Start by asking the children to sit in a circle.

Warm-Up

Say to the children:

We will use ideas from the world of insects for our warm-up!

- **While you are sitting, curl in and out like a pill bug. Try it lying down.**

- Roll onto your back, and imagine you are a bug that is stuck on its back. Move your arms and legs as many ways as you can.

- Roll from side to side like a roly-poly bug, and then bring yourself back up to sitting.

- Inch around the circle like a caterpillar, and end up back where you started.

- Imagine you are a spider, going up and down on your silver thread. Go up and down again, up and down, and finish standing up.

- Let's imagine we are little crickets, and do small bounces as we bend our knees and then straighten them. Now, let's take off from the floor as we do little bouncy jumps.

Large-Motor Skills Practice

Now say to the children:

We are warmed up and ready to do some larger movements across the floor! Let's make a line across the floor, so we can go back and forth while we practice the bigger movements.

As they respond to your movement prompts, the children will travel across the floor together, lined up side by side, with plenty of room between them, and then come back across. Use a drum or tambourine to keep the beat.

- Let's march all the way across the floor together, marching like hard-working ants! Do the same thing coming back across.

- Let's tiptoe like a very quiet bug, all the way across and all the way back.

- Let's walk fast in a zigzag pattern like a spider, all the way across and all the way back.

- Let's hop and jump like a grasshopper as it goes from one blade of grass to another all the way across a field.

- Let's run and swoop like a moth as it flies around a bright light at night. Remember to slow down as you get close to the other side.

- **Let's skip like a water bug across a pond.** Skips are for children ages five and up.

- **Let's leap like a butterfly taking off and landing.** Leaps are for children ages five and up.

Dance Story—*The Little Squeegy Bug*

Gather the children together seated in a circle and read the book *The Little Squeegy Bug*. Ask the children to find home spots throughout the space to begin. Play "Monster Spray" instrumental quietly. Allow each section of the dance story to develop as the children respond to your movement prompts. Say to them:

Squeegy Bug doesn't know what kind of bug he is, so he is going to begin a journey to find out. First he goes to the brook to see Buzzer the Bumblebee. Can you fly like Buzzer? He tells Squeegy Bug to climb to the sky. Can you find a tall cattail and climb to find your silver wings?

Continue the movement using the following prompts at a pace that suits the children:

- **Here come the rain and wind! Can you dance like the storm?**

- **Now you see the caterpillar. How does a caterpillar move?**

- **Visit Haunchy the Spider and his castle of webs. Knock on the door! Walk with Haunchy to the top of the cattail.**

- **Spin silver threads like Haunchy. Try out your new silver wings and fly!**

For this part of the dance, play "Sunscreen" instrumental. Pass out one flashlight or fiber-optic light to each child, and if feasible, turn off the lights. Continue the dance, using these prompts:

- **Reach up in the sky to find a star, and use it as your lantern. Light up the sky, Squeegy the Firefly!**

- **Now take a big bow, fireflies, to end our dance!**

Draw a Squeegy Bug

Collect the flashlights or fiber-optic lights. Bring the children together seated in a circle and say to them:

Now you will draw pictures about the ideas from our dance. I will roll out this long sheet of paper. Please sit down along the edge of the paper while I pass out some crayons. Draw your own squeegy bug— any kind of bug you wish!

If this project is a continuation from Busy Bugs Sessions 1 or 2, tell the children to find the pictures they drew before and draw next to them now.

Presentation Ideas

Busy Bugs Session 3: Squeegy Bugs becomes part of the informal presentation to be performed by the children on the last day of this five-session Busy Bugs activity. If, however, you want to present ideas from this session as a mini-performance, there are several things that would make a fun presentation:

- the warm-up and large-motor skills practice

- the *Little Squeegy Bug* dance story, using the children's drawings of little squeegy bugs as a backdrop

Finish the performance with the children taking another big bow.

For more performance tips, review points one through five and seven, eight, and nine in the list on pages 300–302.

Modifications

One of the advantages of a dance story is that children may participate as much or as little as they are able and willing. A child who is unable to participate in the large-movement portions of this activity can participate with the other children by doing smaller movements in response to the prompts. For example, during Squeegy Bug's journey, the child can stay in one spot and do the smaller movements, such as using arms to fly instead of moving around the space. He can also manipulate the prop while staying in one spot.

Busy Bugs
Session 4: So Many Bugs!

"Busy Bugs Session 4: So Many Bugs!" is inspired by the qualities and characteristics of a variety of bugs. It incorporates a study of opposites through movement, a dance-and-freeze game, and an art project in which the children design and make their own antennae to wear while dancing.

What You Need

☼ a large space

☼ "Kweezletown" instrumental (disc 2, track 27), "Dance S'More" instrumental, and "Bumblebee" instrumental (disc 1, tracks 20 and 14)

☼ antennae made from plastic headbands, pipe cleaners, and large plastic beads

What You Do

Begin with a dance-and-freeze game to music. Have the children find home spots. Say to them:

We will begin today's session with a dance-and-freeze game about different bugs! When you hear the music, you may dance freely around the space. When I stop the music, freeze in the shape of the bug I call out. It could be a grasshopper, a ladybug, a spider, or a butterfly!

Play "Kweezletown" instrumental. Start and stop the music, calling out a different bug each time. Finish the game by asking the children to freeze in the shape of their favorite bug when the music ends.

Continue the activity with a warm-up about different kinds of bugs and how they move. Add ideas and variations you and the children develop as you do the warm-up. Have the children sit in a circle.

Warm-Up

Say to the children:

Let's continue using ideas from the world of insects for our warm-up!

- **While you are sitting, curl in and out like a pill bug. Try it lying down.**

- **Roll onto your back, and imagine you are a bug that is stuck on its back. Move your arms and legs as many ways as you can.**

- **Roll from side to side like a roly-poly bug, and then bring yourself back up to sitting.**

- **Inch around the circle like a caterpillar, and end up back where you started.**

- **Imagine you are a spider, going up and down on your silver thread. Go up and down again, up and down, and finish standing up.**

- **Let's imagine we are little crickets, and do small bounces as we bend our knees and then straighten them. Now let's take off from the floor as we do little bouncy jumps.**

Large-Motor Skills Practice

Now say to the children:

We are warmed up and ready to do some larger movements across the floor! Let's make a line so we can go back and forth while we practice the bigger movements.

As they respond to your movement prompts, the children will travel across the floor together, side by side, with plenty of room between them, and then come back across. Use a drum or tambourine to keep the beat.

- **Let's march all the way across the floor together, marching like hardworking ants! Do the same thing coming back across.**

- Let's tiptoe like a very quiet bug, all the way across and all the way back.

- Let's walk fast in a zigzag pattern like a spider, all the way across and all the way back.

- Let's hop and jump like a grasshopper as it goes from one blade of grass to another, all the way across a field.

- Let's run and swoop like a moth as it flies around a bright light at night. Remember to slow down as you get close to the other side.

- **Let's skip like a water bug across a pond.** Skips are for children ages five and up.

- **Let's leap like a butterfly taking off and landing.** Leaps are for children ages five and up.

Free Dance—Opposites

Ask the children to begin in a home spot, either standing in a circle or spread throughout the large space. Say to them:

This movement game about opposites uses ideas from the insect world. While the music is playing, I will call out the opposites. Stay near your home spot as you dance. Play "Dance S'More" instrumental.

Can you dance high like a bug that flies way up in the sky? Now can you dance low like a bug that burrows in the ground?

Continue the movement using the following prompts at a pace that suits the children:

- **Can you dance slowly like a slow caterpillar? Now can you dance fast like a bumblebee?**

- **Can you dance in a smooth, graceful way like a butterfly, and then can you dance in an uneven, herky-jerky way like a housefly?**

- **Can you dance quietly like a spider, and then loudly like a buzzing mosquito?**

For these next opposites, you may move away from your spot, and dance in the large space.

- **Can you hop small like a little cricket? Now can you hop big like a great big grasshopper?**

- **Can you move around like you have little tiny legs like an itsy-bitsy spider, and then as if you have great big legs like a daddy longlegs?**

- **Can you dance using small movements in your arms and legs like a busy little ant, and then swoop and twirl like a beautiful butterfly, doing big movements with your arms and legs?**

Okay, butterflies, let's land on a leaf and fold our wings. Now we are going to do a quieter activity, and use our imaginations some more.

Draw a Bug

Bring the children together seated in a circle and say to them:

After I roll out this long sheet of paper, you sit down along the edge of it. Now I'll pass out some crayons, and while I do, you think about all of the bugs we have talked about and danced about. Now draw an imaginary bug, with all of your favorite ideas in one bug!

If this project is a continuation from previous Busy Bugs Sessions 1, 2, or 3, tell the children to find the pictures they drew before and draw this one next to the others.

Antennae

Now let's come into a circle. We'll sit and make some antennae to wear for our next dance. You can imagine you are a giant bug, and you are making your own antennae!

Help each child make antennae by twisting pipe cleaners around the plastic headband and decorating the pipe cleaners with beads or any other materials you have on hand.

Free Dance—So Many Bugs!

Now we will try out our antennae! Put them on, and we will do a free dance about bugs, all the ones we danced about earlier in our warm-up exercises and in our game about opposites, and imaginary ones too! You may dance freely in the large space.

Play "Bumblebee" instrumental. When the music ends, have the children finish the dance by doing a big beetle bow. Collect the antennae for use later.

Presentation Ideas

Busy Bugs Session 4: So Many Bugs! becomes part of the informal presentation to be performed by the children on the last day of this five-session Busy Bugs activity. If you want to present ideas from this session as a mini-performance, there are several things that would make a fun presentation:

- the warm-up and large-motor skills practice

- the Opposites free dance and/or the So Many Bugs! free dance, using the children's drawings of bugs as a backdrop

Finish the performance with the children taking another big beetle bow.

For more performance tips, review points one through five and eight and nine in the list on pages 300–302.

Modifications

Have the child who is unable to stand participate in the floor portion of the warm-up. She can help keep the beat by clapping or playing a drum or tambourine during the large-motor skills practice. A child who is not ambulatory can participate in the opposites free dance by staying in one spot, even during the second part, which involves moving about the space. For example, for the prompt "Can you move around like you have little tiny legs like an itsy-bitsy spider, and then as if you have great big legs like a daddy longlegs?" the child can respond by moving her legs in small ways, then using bigger movements, all while seated or lying in one spot. The same applies to the So Many Bugs! free dance. The instructions can be modified so that children who cannot move throughout the space can dance about many different bugs while seated, lying down, or standing in one spot.

Busy Bugs Session 5: Dancing about Bugs for Parents and Friends

· · · · · · · · · · · · · · · · · · ·

"Busy Bugs Session 5: Dancing about Bugs for Parents and Friends" is a review of some of the activities from the previous four sessions, and preparation for an informal performance for an audience. The children will enjoy showing their bug exploration to family, friends, and/or fellow students.

What You Need

☼ Use "Goldie Waltz" instrumental (disc 2, track 24), "Bumblebee" instrumental (disc 1, track 14), "Monster Spray" instrumental, "Sunscreen" instrumental, and "Shakers" instrumental (disc 2, tracks 31, 40, and 36)

☼ pictures of unusual spiders (from session 1); a large black cloth (from session 2; optional), sparkly fabric squares (from session 2); small flashlights or fiber-optic lights (from session 3); headband antennae (from session 4); a drum or a tambourine

What You Do

Begin with a warm-up about different kinds of bugs and how they move. Add ideas and variations you and the children develop as you do the warm-up. Start by asking the children to sit in a circle.

Warm-Up

Say to the children:

We will use ideas from the world of insects for our warm-up!

- **While you are sitting, curl in and out like a pill bug. Try it lying down.**

- **Roll onto your back, and imagine you are a bug that is stuck on its back. Move your arms and legs as many ways as you can.**

- **Roll from side to side like a roly-poly bug, and then bring yourself back up to sitting.**

- **Inch around the circle like a caterpillar, and end up back where you started.**

- **Imagine you are a spider, going up and down on your silver thread. Go up and down again, up and down, and finish standing up.**

- **Let's imagine we are little crickets, and do small bounces as we bend our knees and then straighten them. Now let's take off from the floor as we do little bouncy jumps.**

Large-Motor Skills Practice

Now say to the children:

We are warmed up and ready to do some larger movements across the floor! Let's make a line across the floor so we can go back and forth while we practice the bigger movements.

As they respond to your movement prompts, the children will travel across the floor together, lined up side by side, with plenty of room between them, and then come back across. Use a drum or tambourine to keep the beat.

- **Let's march all the way across the floor together, marching like hard-working ants! Do the same thing coming back across.**

- **Let's tiptoe like a very quiet bug, all the way across and all the way back.**

- **Let's walk fast in a zigzag pattern like a spider, all the way across and all the way back.**

- **Let's hop and jump like a grasshopper as it goes from one blade of grass to another, all the way across a field.**

- **Let's run and swoop like a moth as it flies around a bright light at night. Remember to slow down as you get close to the other side.**

- **Let's skip like a water bug across a pond.** Skips are for children ages five and up.

- **Let's leap like a butterfly taking off and landing.** Leaps are for children ages five and up.

Ask the children which parts of the warm-up and large-motor skills practice they would like to show the audience who will come later in the day to see their presentation. The children may decide they want to show all of the warm-up and large-motor skills activities!

The Presentation

Now it is time to prepare for the performance and then present it to the audience! Here are the steps that you will take to set up and guide the children through the presentation.

1. Prepare the space. Gather all of the props together and arrange them so they are ready for each dance story. Hang the large sheet of bug pictures the children made as a backdrop for the presentation. Arrange chairs for the audience so they face the performance area. Base the number of invitees on the size of your space, allowing plenty of room for the dancers to move and the audience to sit comfortably.

2. Review the order of the performance with the children. About five minutes before it is time for the audience to arrive, ask the children to sit in their spots in the circle. Ask them to remain seated in their spots until the presentation begins.

3. Greet the audience. You can say: **Welcome, family and friends! We have a fun show for you today! We have been studying bugs for these past five days and would like to share many different**

aspects of our exploration with you. The children are seated where they will begin their warm-up.

4. Explain the movement study. You can say: **Before we start, I would like to tell you about our backdrop and our movement explorations. The long sheet of paper hanging as our backdrop, with all of its colorful drawings, is a cumulative study. On each of the first four days, the children added a new bug based on our movement studies and explorations.**

   During our movement activities, we used these pictures of unusual spiders, pictures of the life cycle of a moth or butterfly, the book *The Little Squeegy Bug* by Bill Martin Jr. and Michael Sampson, delightful music by Debbie Clement, and some fun props, such as flashlights and sparkly fabric. Show the audience the various props as you say this. **The best ingredient, and the one we had ready at all times, was our imaginations!**

   We will begin our presentation by showing you our warm-up and large-motor skills exercises. We did these every day to get ready to dance. You will see that everything we do today is about bugs!

5. Begin the performance! Show the audience a few—or, if there is time, all—of the warm-up and large-motor skills activities. If you do not have time to do all of them, then tell the audience the children have chosen their favorite movements to perform. Use a drum or tambourine as accompaniment. When the children have finished, say to the audience: **Now that we are warmed up, we will show you a dance story about the life cycle of a butterfly or moth. The dance story is called "Caterpillars and Cocoons."**

6. Do the first dance story—Caterpillars and Cocoons (from session 2). Say to the children: **Please go to your home spots in the large space and get ready to dance.** The children should use these same home spots to begin both dance stories. When showing this dance story to the audience, use the same movement prompts you used while developing the story with the children. Because the movement is improvised, the dance will be different each time. The children will respond in movement as you tell the story with the prompts. As always, allow enough time for each section of the story to develop.

Use the large black cloth, if available, and sparkly fabric squares, two per child. Finish with the children bowing to the audience, still holding the squares, or butterfly wings. Play "Goldie Waltz" instrumental and "Bumblebee" instrumental while the children dance.

7. Do the next dance story—*The Little Squeegy Bug* (from session 3). Say to the audience: **Our next dance is a story about a little bug who doesn't know what he is, and he goes on a journey. His adventures help him find out what kind of bug he is.**

As with the Caterpillars and Cocoons dance story, use the same movement prompts that were used when developing this dance, and the flashlight props. Children will begin in the same home spots they used in the last dance. They will wear the antennae for this dance. Finish with a big squeegy bug bow. Play "Monster Spray" instrumental and "Sunscreen" instrumental.

8. Finish the performance. To conclude, do the caterpillar conga line from session 2. Briefly describe the dance to the audience. Play "Shakers" instrumental. Line the children up behind you, beat the conga rhythm a few times on your drum or tambourine with the music, or clap your hands, so the children hear the rhythm before they start. Lead the children around the room, still wearing their antennae. Ask them to wave good-bye as they walk by the audience. Use the caterpillar conga line to lead the children out of the performance space, or into the audience, or whatever works best in your space. If you prefer, you can lead them so they end up in a line facing the audience to take one last bow.

9. Thank the audience for coming and the children for sharing their dancing with the audience. If there is time, invite the audience to ask you and the children questions about the five movement-exploration sessions about bugs.

INDEX OF MUSICAL SELECTIONS

ACTIVITIES THAT WORK WELL OUTSIDE

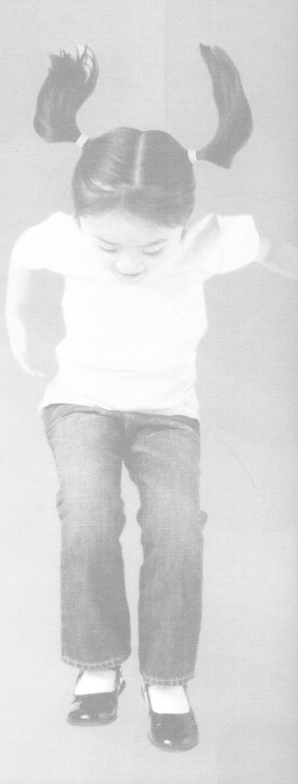

Activity 1: High Five

Activity 2: No-Hands Shake

Activity 3: Our Special Greeting

Activity 4: Morning Rap

Activity 22: Fast and Slow, High and Low

Activity 24: Space Suits

Activity 26: Tightrope Walker

Activity 27: Surprise!

Activity 28: Follow My Footsteps

Activity 54: "Run" Rhymes with "Fun"!

Activity 55: Action Words in English and Spanish

Activity 63: From Top to Bottom

Activity 65: Imagine

Activity 67: I Can

Activity 68: Dance Story – Dinosaur Romp

Activity 73: Parade

Activity 79: Cats and Lions on the Prowl

Activity 80: Fun with Marching

Activity 81: More Fun with Marching

Activity 82: Walk, Trot, Prance, Gallop!

Activity 83: The Dancing Letter "H"

Activity 87: Step, Hop, Skip, Skip, Skip!

Activity 88: Learning to Leap

Activity 89: Opposites

Activity 91: Go and Stop

Activity 93: Straight, Flop

ACTIVITIES THAT REQUIRE A LARGE SPACE

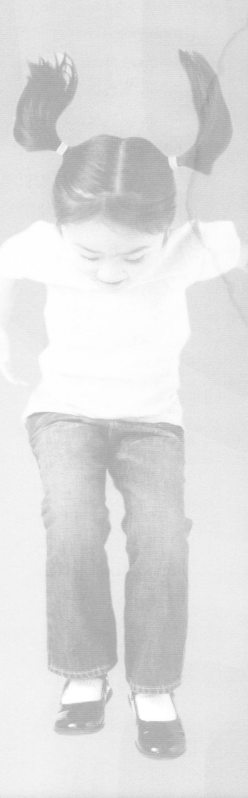

Activity 14: Start Fidgeting!

Activity 22: Fast and Slow, High and Low

Activity 24: Space Suits

Activity 37: Action Alphabet "E" and "F"

Activity 38: Action Alphabet "G"

Activity 44: Action Alphabet "M" and "N"

Activity 45: Action Alphabet "O," "P," and "Q"

Activity 46: Action Alphabet "R"

Activity 50: Action Alphabet "X," "Y," and "Z"

Activity 51: Word Rhythms

Activity 53: The Language of Gestures

Activity 54: "Run" Rhymes with "Fun"!

Activity 55: Action Words in English and Spanish

Activity 59: Move and Freeze

Activity 63: From Top to Bottom

Activity 64: Muscle Mania

Activity 65: Imagine

Activity 66: Dance Story—Baby Birdie Boogie

Activity 67: I Can

Activity 68: Dance Story—Dinosaur Romp

Activity 70: Eating Healthy

Activity 71: Motion in the Ocean

Activity 73: Parade

Activity 74: Dance Story—Digging the Dirt

Activity 75: Grocery Space Trip

Activity 77: Let's Take a Bus Ride

Activity 78: Baby Steps

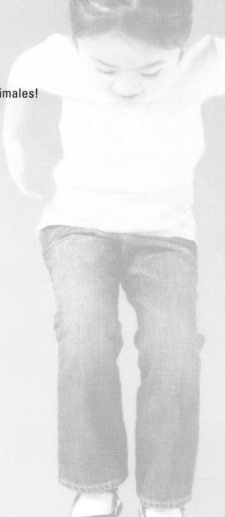

ACTIVITIES ABOUT NATURE—ANIMALS, PLANTS, AND WEATHER

ANIMALS

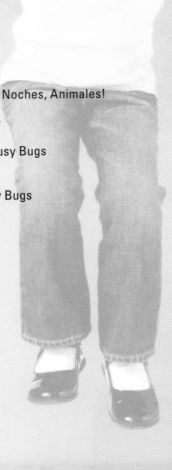

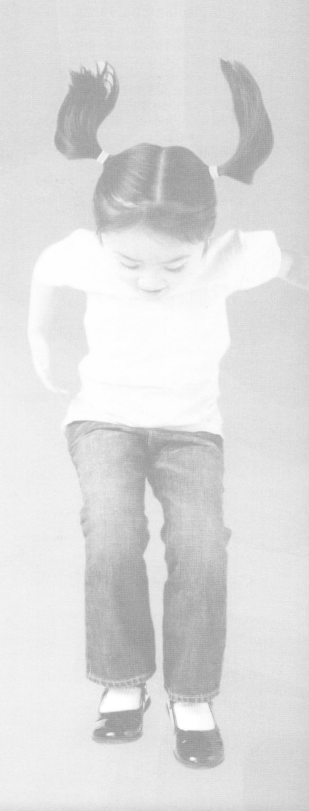

PLANTS

WEATHER

Song Lyrics

DIG, DIG, DIG (CD 1, TRACK 1)
I like to dig, dig, dig in the dirt.
I like to dig, dig, dig in the dirt.
When the sun is in the sky and the clouds
    go rolling by,
I like to dig, dig, dig in the dirt.
I like to dig, dig, dig in the dirt.
That's how the veggies grow, you plant
    the seeds down low.
I like to dig, dig, dig in the dirt.
I like to dig, dig, dig in the dirt.

When the sun is in the sky and the bees
    go buzzing by,
I like to dig, dig, dig in the dirt.
I like to dig, dig, dig in the dirt.
That's how the veggies grow, you plant
    them in a row.
I like to dig, dig, dig in the dirt.
I like to dig, dig, dig in the dirt.

When the sun is in the sky and the ants
    go marching by,
I like to dig, dig, dig in the dirt.
I like to dig, dig, dig in the dirt.
That's how the veggies grow, you water
    them and they go.
I like to dig, dig, dig in the dirt.
I like to dig, dig, dig in the dirt.

When the sun is in the sky and the worms
    go wiggling by,
I like to dig, dig, dig in the dirt.
I like to dig, dig, dig in the dirt.
That's how the veggies grow, you weed
    them with a hoe.
I like to dig, dig, dig in the dirt.
I like to dig, dig, dig in the dirt.

When the sun is in the sky and my song
    goes singing by,
I like to dig, dig, dig in the dirt.
I like to dig, dig, dig in the dirt.
That's how the veggies grow, you harvest
    before the snow.

I like to dig, dig, dig in the dirt.
I like to dig, dig, dig in the dirt.

When the sun is in the sky and the day
    goes drifting by,
I like to dig, dig, dig in the dirt.
I like to dig, dig, dig in the dirt.
That's how the flowers grow, pretty colors
    that I know.
I like to dig, dig, dig in the dirt.
I like to dig, dig, dig in the dirt.
I like to dig, dig, dig in the dirt.
I like to dig, dig, dig!

DINOSAUR ROMP (CD 1, TRACK 2)
It's time to do the dinosaur romp.
Wade with me in a prehistoric swamp.
Turn on your imagination.
Join me on the dinosaur station.
Look across your dinosaur map.
Let's get movin' to our prehistoric rap!

Stomp your feet now very loud.
Brontosaurus was mighty proud.
Travelin' through the prehistoric swamp,
Join me in the brontosaurus stomp!
Stomp, stomp, stomp, stomp.
Stomp, stomp, stomp, stomp!

Flap your wings now very soft.
Pterodactyl could fly aloft.
Feel the beat of the prehistoric rap.
Join me in the pterodactyl flap!
Flap, flap, flap, flap.
Flap, flap, flap, flap!
Join me in the brontosaurus stomp!
Stomp, stomp, stomp, stomp.
Stomp, stomp, stomp, stomp!

Chomp your teeth now very clean.
Tyrannosaurus was very mean.
Travelin' through the prehistoric swamp,
Join me in the tyrannosaurus chomp!
Chomp, chomp, chomp, chomp.

Chomp, chomp, chomp, chomp!
Join me in the pterodactyl flap!
Flap, flap, flap, flap.
Flap, flap, flap, flap!
Join me in the brontosaurus stomp!
Stomp, stomp, stomp, stomp.
Stomp, stomp, stomp, stomp.
Stomp, stomp, stomp, stomp!

We're all done with the dinosaur romp.
Let's wade back out of the prehistoric swamp.
Turn off your imagination.
We are leavin' the dinosaur station.
Put away your dinosaur map.
We're all done with the dinosaur rap!

EATING HEALTHY (CD 1, TRACK 3)
Chorus
Eating healthy, being healthy,
That's the choice for me.
Eating healthy, being healthy,
Yes, ma'am, yessiree!
Eating healthy, being healthy,
That's how I will choose.
Eating healthy, being healthy,
I'll be healthy, you'll be healthy.
Help me spread the news!

Repeat chorus.

Green beans, crunchy carrots,
Broc-broc-broccoli.
I choose my yummy veggies very happily!
Tomatoes, cauliflower,
sweet potatoes, beets.
So many colors of veggies,
and all are good for me!

Repeat chorus.

All the peppers, spinach, okra,
Zu-zu-zucchini.
I choose my yummy veggies very happily!
Bok choy, brussels sprouts, asparagus, and peas.
So many colors of veggies,
and all are good for me!

Repeat chorus.

FOLLOW GAME (CD 1, TRACK 4)
It's time to sing and play the follow game.
Follow me and move just the same.
Come follow me, and move the same.
It's time to play the follow game.
It's time to sing and play the follow game.
Follow me and move just the same.
Come follow me, and move the same.
It's time to play the follow game.

Let's get started with the shoulder shrug.
Shrug your shoulder sweet.
Feel the beat! It's really neat!
With the shoulder shrug.
And then you move . . .
And then you stop—
For a great big hug.
Now we're finished with the shoulder shrug.

Show your stuff with the muscle mug.
Pump your muscles sweet.
Feel the beat! It's really neat!
With the muscle mug.
And then you move . . .
And then you stop—
For a great big hug.
Now we're finished with muscle mug.

Let's move onto the 'squito bug.
Buzz your fingers sweet.
Feel the beat! It's really neat!
With the 'squito bug.
And then you move . . .
And then you stop—
For a great big hug.
Now we're finished with the 'squito bug.

This is harder, try the wiper wug.
Swish your wiper sweet.
Feel the beat! It's really neat!
With the wiper wug.
And then you move . . .
And then you stop—
For a great big hug.
Now we're finished with the wiper wug!

Now we're finished with the follow game.
You followed me and moved just the same.
You followed me, and moved the same.

We're finished with the follow game.
Now we're finished with the follow game.
You followed me and moved just the same.
You followed me, and moved the same.
We're finished with the follow game.

GROCERY SPACE TRIP (CD 1, TRACK 5)

Time to go to the grocery store,
The grocery store,
The grocery store.
Time to go to the grocery store.
We'll buy fresh fruit and a whole lot more!

Take a ride in the shopping cart,
The shopping cart,
The shopping cart.
Take a ride in the shopping cart.
That's my very favorite part!

Pretend my cart is a rocket ship,
A rocket ship,
A rocket ship.
Pretend my cart is a rocket ship.
Get ready now for my space trip!

I'm flying now through outer space,
Outer space,
Outer space.
I'm flying now through outer space,
Headed for the astronaut base!

I like to travel through the stars,
Through the stars,
Through the stars.
I like to travel through the stars,
Looking at Jupiter and Mars!

We landed safely on the moon,
On the moon,
On the moon.
We landed safely on the moon,
Headed back home now very soon!

We're going through the checkout line,
The checkout line,
The checkout line.
We're going through the checkout line.
Our trip to the grocery store was mighty fine!

HAPPY FACE (CD 1, TRACK 6)

Put on your happy face.
Beam your smile throughout this place.
Put on your happy face right now.
Draw a smile from ear to ear.
Brighten up and spread good cheer.
Put on your happy face right now.

I'll show you how!
I'll show you how!
Put on your happy face.
Beam your smile throughout this place.
Put on your happy face right now!

Put on your happy face.
Radiate good will and grace.
Put on your happy face with me.
Draw a smile from ear to ear.
Brighten up and spread good cheer.
Put on your happy face with me.
Tee-hee-hee-hee!
Tee-hee-hee-hee!
Put on your happy face.
Radiate good will and grace.
Put on your happy face with me.

Put on your happy face.
Shine your smile throughout this space.
Put on your happy face, indeed.
Draw a smile from ear to ear.
Brighten up and spread good cheer.
Put on your happy face, indeed!
And you'll succeed!
And you'll succeed!
Put on your happy face.
Shine your smile throughout this place.
Put on your happy face, indeed.

Put on your happy face.
Be a winner in the smiling race.
Put on your happy face today.
Draw a smile from ear to ear.
Brighten up and spread good cheer.
Put on your happy face today.
Hip-hip-hooray!
Hip-hip-hooray!
Put on your happy face.
Be a winner in the smiling race.
Put on your happy face today.
Put on your happy face today.
Put on your happy face today.
Hip-hip-hooray!

JAMBO: HELLO (CD 1, TRACK 7)
Jambo, jambo, how are you?
I learned Swahili, so can you!
Jambo, jambo, how are you?
I learned Swahili, so can you!

Children in Africa smile when they sing.
All of those smiles mean the same thing.
Children round the world all smile when they sing.
All of those smiles mean the same thing!

Hola, hola, how are you?
I learned some Spanish, so can you!
Hola, hola, how are you?
I learned some Spanish, so can you!

Children in Mexico smile when they sing.
All of those smiles mean the same thing.
Children round the world all smile when they sing.
All of those smiles mean the same thing!

Guten Tag, Guten Tag, how are you?
I learned some German, so can you!
Guten Tag, Guten Tag, how are you?
I learned some German, so can you!

Children in Germany smile when they sing.
All of those smiles mean the same thing.
Children round the world all smile when they sing.
All of those smiles mean the same thing!

Bonjour, bonjour, how are you?
I learned some French and so can you!
Bonjour, bonjour, how are you?
I learned some French and so can you!

Children in France all smile when they sing.
All of those smiles mean the same thing.
Children round the world all smile when they sing.
All of those smiles mean the same thing!

Konnichiwa, konnichiwa, how are you?
I learned Japanese, so can you!
Konnichiwa, konnichiwa, how are you?
I learned Japanese, so can you!

Children in Japan all smile when they sing.
All of those smiles mean the same thing.
Children round the world all smile when they sing.
All of those smiles mean the same thing!

Children round the world all smile when they sing.
All of those smiles mean the same thing!

JUMPIN' JIMINY (CD 1, TRACK 8)
Boys and girls from far and wide,
Here's a game we can play inside.
Stand up straight like a pogo stick,
Feet together to do this trick.
Now breathe real slow,
'Cause here we go!

Chorus A
Jumpin' jiminy jamboree,
Jubilation, jubilee.
Jazzy jesters joyfully,
Jubilation, jubilee.
Jumpin' jiminy jamboree,
Jubilation, jubilee.
Jazzy jesters joyfully,
Jubilation, jubilee.
Now breathe real slow,
'Cause here we go!

Chorus B
Freezing, frozen,
Fantastically.
Funsters, frigid, fraggledy-free.
Breathing deeply,
You and me.
Falling, falling,
Now set free!

Repeat chorus A and chorus B.

Girls and boys from wide and far,
Our game's done, you were a star.
Sit back down upon your seat.
Feet now quiet, nice and neat.
Now breathe real slow.
Now we're ready to go!

"LITTLE BIRDIE" (CD 1, TRACK 9)

Baby birdie, little baby birdie,
Fly up high, fly up high.
Baby birdie, little baby birdie,
In the sky, in the sky.

Repeat.

Baby birdie, little baby birdie,
Fly down low, fly down low.
Baby birdie, little baby birdie,
Fly real slow, fly real slow.

Repeat.

Fly, baby bird, fly,
High in the sky,
Watch it go by, baby bird.

Baby birdie, little baby birdie,
Tweet tweet tweet, tweet tweet tweet.
Baby birdie, little baby birdie,
Sounds so sweet, sounds so sweet.

Repeat.

Baby birdie, little baby birdie,
In the nest, in the nest.
Baby birdie, little baby birdie,
Take a rest, take a rest.

Repeat.

MONKEY FUN (CD 1, TRACK 10)
Monkey none, monkey one,
Now let's have some monkey fun!

Monkey two, monkey three,
Let's all climb in the monkey tree!

Monkey four, monkey five,
Join me in some monkey jive!

Monkey six, monkey seven,
Jump up and down like monkey heaven!

Monkey eight, monkey nine,
Act like monkeys mighty fine!

Monkey nine, monkey eight,
Let's all do the monkey skate!

Monkey seven, monkey six,
Show me all your monkey tricks!

Monkey five, monkey four,
Raise the roof and dance some more!

Monkey three, monkey two,
Do the monkey how-de-do!

Monkey one, monkey none,
Now we're done with monkey fun!

Repeat verses.

Everybody have a seat,
Sit back down and feel the beat!
Everybody sit back down,
Hear the monkeys go to town!

PATTERN SONG (CD 1, TRACK 11)
Here we go, it's a pattern song.
Listen and watch, and play along!
We will start with an easy one.
Listen and watch, and have some fun!

Are you ready? It's a pattern song.
Listen and watch, 'cause you belong!

Knees, tap, knees, tap, knees, tap, knees, tap.
Knees, tap, knees, tap, knees, tap, knees . . . tap!

Head, ear, ear, head, ear, ear, head, ear, ear,
     head, ear, ear.
Head, ear, ear, head, ear, ear, head, ear, ear, head . . .
     ear, ear!

Stomp, stomp, clap, stomp, stomp, clap, stomp,
     stomp, clap, stomp, stomp, clap.
Stomp, stomp, clap, stomp, stomp, clap, stomp,
     stomp, clap, stomp, stomp . . . clap!

Hip, hip, zoom, zoom, hip, hip, zoom, zoom, hip, hip,
     zoom, zoom, hip, hip, zoom, zoom.
Hip, hip, zoom, zoom, hip, hip, zoom, zoom, hip, hip,
     zoom, zoom, hip, hip . . . zoom, zoom!

Wrist, wrist, chin-chin-chin, wrist, wrist, chin-chin-
     chin, wrist, wrist, chin-chin-chin, wrist, wrist,
     chin-chin-chin.
Wrist, wrist, chin-chin-chin, wrist, wrist, chin-chin-
     chin, wrist, wrist, chin-chin-chin, wrist, wrist . . .
     chin-chin-chin!

Now we're done with the pattern song.
You listened, you watched, you played along.
We got started with an easy one.
You listened, you watched, we had some fun!

And now we're done!

SUNSCREEN (CD 1, TRACK 12)

Chorus
The sun is out.
Let's give a shout—hey!
Hip-hip-hooray, it's a sunny day.

Repeat chorus.

It's time to rub on sunscreen
To keep you safe from harm.
It's time to rub on sunscreen.
Please remember my . . . arm!

Repeat chorus twice.

It's time to rub on sunscreen.
Please don't make me beg.
It's time to rub on sunscreen.
Please remember my . . . leg!

Repeat chorus twice.

It's time to rub on sunscreen.
Help me, will you please?
It's time to rub on sunscreen.
Please remember my . . . knees!

Repeat chorus twice.

It's time to rub on sunscreen.
Now you've got the knack.
It's time to rub on sunscreen.
Please remember my . . . back!

Repeat chorus twice.

It's time to rub on sunscreen.
Rub it over here.
It's time to rub on sunscreen.
Please remember my . . . ear!

Repeat chorus twice.

It's time to rub on sunscreen.
I'm starting to smell sweet.
It's time to rub on sunscreen.
Please remember my . . . feet!

Repeat chorus twice.

We've rubbed on all the sunscreen.
We're ready for the sun.
We've rubbed on all the sunscreen.
Let's go outside and have . . . fun!

Repeat chorus twice.

All music, lyrics, and arrangements are under copyright by Debbie Clement. All rights reserved. Published by exclusive arrangement with Debbie Clement.
All songs were written and performed by Debbie Clement.
All songs and instrumentals were arranged by Tom Martin.
All songs and instrumentals were recorded at Amerisound Studios, Columbus, Ohio.
All songs and instrumentals were engineered by Dan Green. Background vocals and sound effects were also provided by Dan Green.
All studio guitar, mandolin, and banjo were performed by Larry Cook.

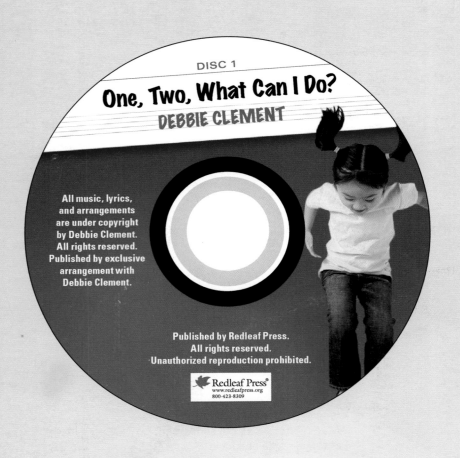

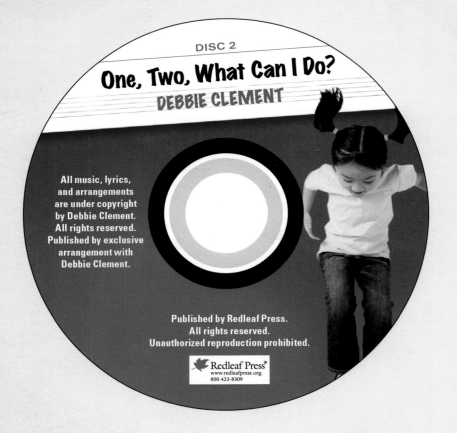